Nothing written in th
for sound medical ad
are advised to consult your health care professional before
making any changes in diet. Application of the information
and recommendations in this book are undertaken at the
individual's own risk. The author did his best to make sure
all sources used were accurate and current. The author and
publisher disclaim all liability in connection with the use of
the information presented herein.

Street Smart Vegan. © 2010 by Jay Wesley Anderson & Brevity
Holdings LLC. First Edition

All Rights Reserved. Except as permitted under the U.S.
Copyright Act of 1976, this book may not be reproduced in
whole or in part, in any form or by any means, electronic
or mechanical, including photocopying, recording, or by
any information storage and retrieval system now known
or hereafter invented, without written permission from the
publisher.

Brevity Holdings LLC
2153 Wealthy St.
Suite #112
Grand Rapids, MI 49506

Printed in the United States of America

ISBN 978-0-9824985-0-7 (pbk.)

Cover and book design by Heather DeGroff
Edited by Mary Clarke

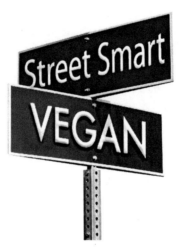

A Simple System for Going Vegan

By Jay Wesley Anderson

Printed on paper from a certified sustainable forest.

Contents At A Glance

Author's Welcome 9

Chapter 1: Crisis Meets Opportunity 11
  Consumption 12
  What Is A Vegan? 13
  Why Be Vegan? 13
  Einstein Was No Dummy 14
  Putting the Puzzle Pieces Together 16

Chapter 2: A Simple Process for Going Vegan 17
  Step 1: Acknowledge The Overwhelming Benefits 18
  Step 2: Decide To Commit 18
  Step 3: Enjoy The Process 19
  It's Time To Get Excited 19
  Make the Transition As Gradual As You Want 19

Chapter 3: Being Street Smart With Your pH 20
  Are You Acidic Or Alkaline? 22
  The "Food Pyramid?" 23
  Antioxidants: Your Best Defense 24
  The Most Powerful Source Of
    Antioxidants On Earth 24
  Food Ingredients To Avoid 26
  Great Sweetener Alternatives 29
  MSG Goes Incognito 29
  Keep Your pH Eyes Open 31

Chapter 4: Dairy Is A Con 32
- Osteoporosis 33
- Absorbing Calcium 34
- Dairy = Suffering 35
- Unwanted Results Of Increased Milk Production 36
- Dairy Alternatives 38

Chapter 5: Meat Is Dead Energy 39
- Bio-accumulation Of Toxins 40
- The Protein Frenzy...Is It Legitimate? 41
- Is Too Much Protein Bad? 42
- You Don't Even Need Any Extra Cholesterol 42
- Meat Alternatives 43
- P.S. Want More Energy? 44

Chapter 6: Clean Water Is Your Buddy 46
- Water Brings You Vitality 47
- Your Body Will Let You Know 48
- Salt Is Essential 49
- The Grim Tale Of Tap Water 50
- Consistent Poison In Small Amounts 52
- Getting Clean Water 54

Chapter 7: Interview With A Vegan Mother 55
- What Made You Choose A Vegan Diet? 56

Has The Vegan Diet Interfered With
Your Child's Growth Rate? 58

Are There Any Affirmations That
You Use While Cooking? 61

Taco Recipe From A Vegan Mom 63

Build Your Vegan Taco 65

Quick Links To Recipe Products 66

Chapter 8: Adrenaline, Not For Consumption! 67

Not So Nice 68

Eye To Eye 69

Chapter 9: How To Give Away A Leather Coat 70

Chapter 10: Human Anatomy Tells No Lie 72

Digestion 73

Tools Of The Trade 73

The Intestines Of A Carnivore 74

You've Got A Lot Of Guts 74

Fiber Is Your Friend 75

Chapter 11: Best Thing You Can Do For The Planet 77

Global Warming: What Is It? 78

Numbers Speak Louder Than Words 79

A Planet In Need Of Efficiency 79

The Big Picture 80

The Wrath Of The Livestock Sector 80
Population Growth 82
Each Person's Ecological "Footprint" 82
How To Be Sure You're Buying Organic 83
Why Is Organic Produce Better? 84
How Much Has The Earth Actually Warmed Up? ... 84

Chapter 12: Call To Action 86
Empowering Solutions 87

Chapter 13: A Vegan Day 88
How To Use This Chapter 89
Good Morning 90
Feel The Energy From This Tasty Green Shake 91
How To Locate These Ingredients 92
Why The "Green Drink" Is Awesome 92
Breakfast 93
Lunch Is The New Breakfast 94
Tasty Wraps 94
Remember The Daily Large Salad 95
Why To Use A Generous Amount Of Herbs 95
Having Lunch In A Hurry?
    Take This Sandwich With You 96
Anytime, Take-Along Snacks 96
The Home-Made, Money-Saving Hummus Recipe ... 98
Enjoy Low Sugar Fruits 98

Don't Feel Like Cooking? 99
Afternoon Alkalizing 100
The Dinner Of A Multi-Tasker 100
Being Vegan And Getting Vitamin B-12 101
What Happens If You Fall Off The Vegan Bus? 102

Chapter 14: 3 Common Mistakes New Vegans Make ... 104
    Common Mistake #1: Over-Extending
        A "Lazy Vegan" Phase 105
    Common Mistake #2: Spending Time
        In A Vegan "Bubble" 106
    Common Mistake #3: Not Meeting
        New Vegan Friends 107

Chapter 15: Vegan Road Trips 108

Chapter 16: Social Outings Surrounding Food 111
    Going Out To Eat 112
    Ordering A Drink 113
    Ordering A Meal 113
    You Just Blew Your Cover! 114
    Prepare To Answer These Questions 114
    Speaking On Behalf Of The Vegan Lifestyle 115
    Easy Table Conversation Transitioning 116
    Final Remarks 116

5 Bonus Vegan Recipes 117

A Lazy Vegan Breakfast 118

Traveling Sandwiches 118

Fresh And Energizing Salad 119

The Revive Wrap 119

Berries On A Boat 120

Sources Consulted 122

Endnotes 129

AUTHOR'S WELCOME

When you spot a detour sign on a road, you realize the old way of going is under construction. The old way is being fixed because it's no longer producing functional or acceptable results for those passing through.

This book is a detour sign. How we think about food is under construction. We need safe passage to our destination of good health. This book is here to help you align yourself with healthy, acceptable results.

After years of being misinformed, tired, and unhealthy myself, it's been a blessing to locate this information. It's been a fun detour. I'm happy to share it with you.

Learning about and enjoying vegan foods has been the ultimate intoxicating privilege. The energy that comes from a vegan diet can amplify daily progress, giving you more energy to enrich your life and the lives of others. You won't feel drained from digesting foods like meat and dairy that are simply too potent.

This book doesn't contain all there is to know about health and nutrition. I'm not a nutritionist or a health guru. I'm just a guy who has sifted through plenty of information and misinformation and I'm fascinated enough to not shut up about it.

That said, I suggest you embrace any curious urge to do your own research and seek expert advise from health professionals if necessary.

I'm excited for you. The fact that you are reading this right now indicates that you are curious about making changes that will add to your quality of life. Don't worry what other people think about a vegan diet, the proof will reside in how you feel. And if you look great because you are glowing with vibrant health, all the better!

For me, this journey began on the unforgettable day I was introduced to the irresistible benefits of being vegan. I started asking questions like, "Why is our country so sick?"

Between researching and talking to experts, my findings were compelling enough to push me to write and tell others in a simple way. I write to diffuse the insane amount of clutter and misinformation people find on their road to better health. I write because the environmental future of this planet gains hope as the vegan movement grows.

What started out as a gradual vegan transformation has gained consistency over time. The process continues to be an educational trip as the detour meanders.

— Jay Wesley Anderson

1) CRISIS MEETS OPPORTUNITY

"If anyone wants to save the planet, all they have to do is just stop eating meat. That's the single most important thing you can do."
– *Sir Paul McCartney*

Perhaps more than any point in history, the world is demanding that we change. The economic funk, environmental problems, and disease statistics are really just feedback signals telling us, "Hey, maybe it's time to think about a better approach, maybe it's time to reinvent ourselves."

If we want to give the planet hope for a healthy and prosperous future, we must increase our efficiency at the most basic level, the way we eat. Jean Mayer, a Harvard nutritionist, estimated that reducing meat production in the U.S. by 10 percent would make available an amount of grain to feed 60 million people!

A growing tribe of vegans spreading the good word is the answer. The world is waiting for a lifestyle like this to *explode* in numbers.

CONSUMPTION

Per capita meat consumption rose by 40 percent in the United States between 1961 and 2002.[1] That's a very sudden change if we consider how long humans have been around. I credit this rise to the meat industry's brilliant marketing. Good payday for them, right? Unfortunately, avoidable diseases are the paired result.

Misinformation has been a huge player. We've simply been fed misleading information about how much protein our bodies need and where the best sources of calcium can be found. This misinformation is unacceptable and will be dealt with in Chapters 4 and 5.

Could the missing keystone for a functionally sustainable planet be a change in how the majority of people choose to eat? Given the exponential human population growth we are experiencing, it's important to take a serious look at this question.

WHAT IS A VEGAN?

Vegans don't eat meat, fish, poultry, dairy, or eggs. It's pronounced *"VEE-gun."* The meaning of *vegetarian* has a little more play to it. Some vegetarians might feast on dairy and eggs, where as a vegan consumes no animal products at all.

WHY BE A VEGAN?

If you understand "the why," making the transition to a vegan diet will be more meaningful for you. Here are the 3 pillars that hold up "the why."

Pillar 1 - Increasing Your Overall Health.

By not consuming animal products, vegans have a

better chance of side-stepping many preventable diseases like cancer. The quality of energy delivered by vegan foods can increase your quality of life.

Pillar 2 - *Leaving A Lighter Eco-Footprint*.

The production of animal products is harsher on the environment than you might think. Imagine acres and acres of rainforest being converted into grazing pastures. That's just a glimpse of the devastation brought on by the livestock sector. You'll see in Chapter 11 how going vegan is the best thing you can do for the planet.

Pillar 3 - *Living A Compassionate Lifestyle*.

Since the methods used to produce animal products are out of sight, they are often out of mind. The vast majority of the animal industry runs on profits, not ethics. Vegans choose to boycott the mistreatment of animals.

EINSTEIN WAS NO DUMMY!

Some of the brightest minds in History were vegetarian, or perhaps what we now call vegan. Among them were Albert Einstein, Leonardo da Vinci, Thomas Edison, Ben Franklin, Mahatma Gandhi, Sir Isaac Newton, Plato, Socrates, Charles Darwin, Henry David Thoreau, and Vincent Van

Gogh.[2] That's one stunning list of champion contributors!

If you are currently a vegan or vegetarian, you're not alone. Here's a brief list of athletes, rockers, public figures, and actors you've probably heard of: Fiona Apple, Christina Applegate, Casey Affleck, Bob Barker, Kim Basinger, Angela Bassett, Orlando Bloom, Christie Brinkley, Pierce Broson, Deepak Chopra, Chelsea Clinton, David Duchovny, Clint Eastwood, Shannon Elizabeth, Melssa Etheridge, Corey Feldman, Peter Gabriel, Richard Gere, Woody Harrelson, Dustin Hoffman, Desmond Howard, Mick Jagger, Casey Kasem, Anthony Kiedis, Lenny Kravitz, Dennis Kucinich, Annie Lennox, Phil Lesh, Kenny Loggins, Tobey Maquire, Paul McCartney, Ian McKellen, Natalie Merchant, Moby, Demi Moore, Joe Namath, Martina Navratilova, Olivia Newton-John, Stevie Nicks, Joaquin Phoenix, Natalie Portman, Prince, Bonnie Raitt, Claudia Schiffer, Steven Seagal, Alicia Silverstone, Ringo Starr, Julia Stiles, Tina Turner, Shania Twain, Liv Tyler, Eddie Vedder, Keenen Ivory Wayans, Vanessa Williams, Weird Al Yankovic, and Thom Yorke,[2] These people certainly aren't lacking the energy needed to accomplish amazing results in their respective fields.

PUTTING THE PUZZLE PIECES TOGETHER

If you look long enough, you can find diet philosophies that vouch for almost anything. Then you might find recommendations totally against what you previously found. How do you know what's true? Embrace doing your own research and experimenting to arrive at a lifestyle that puts the puzzle together for you.

If you're not getting the healthy results you want and your body is giving you feedback in the form of a dis-ease, maybe it's time to change your approach. Maybe it's time to reinvent yourself until you feel positive feedback. Are you paying attention to the feedback you are getting? Is your current approach working for you?

"Street smart" as a metaphor works well. It means using common sense to make quick decisions that will increase chances of not only surviving, but thriving. The British Medical Association confirmed that vegetarians have lower rates of obesity, coronary heart disease, high blood pressure, large bowel disorders, cancers, gall stones, and lower levels of cholesterol.[3] *Vegans* are the underrated underdogs that score big on the health charts.

2) A SIMPLE (3 STEP) PROCESS FOR GOING VEGAN

"Being vegan helped me realize I can say and do what I believe is right. That's powerful. Nothing's changed my life more. I feel better about myself as a person, being conscious and responsible for my actions and I lost weight and my skin cleared up and I got bright eyes and I just became stronger and healthier and happier. Can't think of anything better in the world to be but vegan."
– *Alicia Silverstone*

STEP 1: ACKNOWLEDGE THE OVERWHELMING BENEFITS

Your decision to go vegan means you will be leaving a significantly lighter environmental footprint. It feels good to boycott the livestock sector which is literally the worst polluter of all!

You'll be enjoying vegan foods that will give your body all the nutrition it needs. Plus, you will have additional peace of mind knowing that vegan foods are naturally cholesterol free.

You can rest assured knowing that you are eating cruelty-free foods. Being a conscious consumer feels awesome!

STEP 2: DECIDE TO COMMIT

Decide to take action and be in control of your health. This is a far more empowering approach than being in position of re-action when disease knocks at your door.

You'll be surprised how easy and enjoyable it is to maintain a few daily consumption routines that are good for your pH.

This means including alkalizing foods in your diet like leafy green salads, and the "Green Drink" featured in Chapter 13.

STEP 3: ENJOY THE PROCESS

Embrace the detour. Whether it's a new vegan dish you are tasting for the first time, or one of your standby vegan recipes, simply appreciating the food in front of you will make it that much more enjoyable.

ITS TIME TO GET EXCITED!

You've left behind foods that were holding you back from reaching your highest potential energy levels. And guess what? As a vegan, your daily consumption choices now have a solid purpose. Why?

Your consumption choices will be making a measurable difference by leaving a lighter environmental footprint. That's exciting! Feel good about that.

MAKE THE TRANSITION AS GRADUAL AS YOU WANT

Remember, change requires flexibility. If you need to employ the "One Day At A Time" approach at the beginning, do it.

3) BEING STREET SMART WITH YOUR pH

"I've seen people who no longer require insulin injections for their diabetes. People whose aches and pains disappeared. Even people who had been diagnosed with cancer whose tumors vanished and who were pronounced cancer free." [4]
– *Dr. Robert O. Young, "The pH Miracle"*

If you're currently sick or not feeling well, there's always hope. The human body is capable of amazing things if it's given a chance. From what I've read and experienced, the most important thing to pay attention to is eating foods that will keep the pH of the blood slightly alkaline. The human body is complex. Knowing how to keep your pH level in check is the most simple and effective approach to wellness. So what's pH all about?

pH refers to the *acid : alkaline* ratio. It's also called *acid : base* ratio. Basic and alkaline mean the same thing.

Ever had to test the pH of a swimming pool? Our bodies have a pH too. Just like the pool, we don't want our body's pH level to get out of control. If it does, the funk sets in.

Dr. Robert Young and his wife Shelley have done amazing work in their book *The pH Miracle*. I recommend this book to anyone who's really trying to figure out optimal health. If you visit pHmiracleliving.com, you can view alkalizing recipes and sign up to receive emails about fascinating health information. *The pH Miracle* is like my bible. I consult the book about twice a week to figure out the pH of foods I'm eating. I lend it to friends who are feeling crummy.

ARE YOU ACIDIC OR ALKALINE?

Our blood needs to be slightly alkaline.[5] According to Dr. Young, "Overacidity interferes with life itself. It is at the root of all sickness and disease."[6] Dr. Young confirms that meat, eggs, dairy, yeast products, grains, fermented foods, artificial sweeteners, sugars, alcohol, coffee, chocolate, black tea, and sodas are ALL acidifying.

If that list contains all the foods you're currently conditioned to love, don't worry! By keeping acidifying foods to a minimum, you will be rewarded by feeling better. Remember, nothing tastes as good as vitality feels. This can be a gradual transition.

Dr. Young recommends that 80 percent of your diet should come from alkalizing foods. This is a visual, not a caloric or weight, measurement. Vegetables are the alkalizing answer. They help restore your pH.[7]

How do you feel after you eat an amazing salad with lots of leafy greens? It feels good, right? That's because vegetables are alive with energy and beneficial enzymes. Feeling the energy benefits of alkalizing foods puts acidifying foods in their second-rate place.

For fun, let's rewind back to a typical college morning, way before I knew anything about pH. Hung-over from boozing it up the night before, I'd wake up with a cup of coffee with cream and sugar. What awaited for breakfast at the cafeteria? Eggs, toast, bacon, and hash browns. I'd top it off with a glass of sugary orange juice. Not exactly a pH recipe for success. No wonder my spirits were consistently low and my health was suffering.

Now I make sure my pH is where it needs to be by consciously alkalizing. Here's a short list of alkalizing foods that I employ daily: pure soy lecithin granules, liquid chlorophyll, a green drink powder that contains wheat grass, aloe, and flax seed oil. With some research and experimenting, you may find more potentials that work for you. In Chapter 13 you'll find out how and when to mix the above ingredients into green goodness drink of your own.

THE "FOOD PYRAMID?"

The recommendations given by the food pyramid have an overall acidic effect on the body.[8] Is it any surprise that people in the United States are so obese and sick? Not really, considering that most people trust the food pyramid and consume accordingly. Realizing that the status quo foods you may have learned to love are wrecking havoc on your pH is a good first step to becoming alkaline.

So what should we think about our tax dollars funding a Food and Drug Administration that sets us up to fail with a bunk food pyramid? It is a hard pill to swallow. But enough of the whining protest. The misinformation stops here.

ANTIOXIDANTS

Red wine contains antioxidants. Vegetables do too. What are antioxidants? Antioxidants work to cancel out harmful free radicals that can damage body cells.[9] What if the food or beverage of choice has an acidic repercussion on your pH, like red wine? Then it's time to find a more street smart source of antioxidants!

THE MOST POWERFUL SOURCES OF ANTIOXIDANTS ON EARTH

Raw chocolate has over 300 nutritional compounds and is among the richest sources of antioxidants on earth.[10] I'm not talking about the sugar spike-then-crash from a processed Hershey's chocolate bar.

Cornell University scientists found that raw chocolate has far more antioxidants than red wine or green tea.[11] Sunfood Nutrition sells an 8-ounce package of organic raw chocolate nibs for about $13. Information on the package details that raw chocolate has 20 times more antioxidants than red wine and 30 times more than green tea! All that, and it makes you feel euphoric.

Raw chocolate is also an abundant source of magnesium. Magnesium is an energy mineral and all-important electrolyte that is good for heart function.[12] How about buying your true love the real thing next Valentine's Day?

On the Oxygen Radical Absorbance Capacity scale that measures the antioxidant magnitude in foods, goji berries score big.[13] Goji berries are 8 times more powerful in antioxidants than raisins and they're over 25 times more robust with antioxidants than broccoli.[14] Goji berries have also been called an anti-aging food.[15]

Guess what? They taste awesome. You can find out more about goji berries and raw chocolate at sunfood.com.

FOOD INGREDIENTS TO AVOID

There must be a reason why Europe and Canada have banned the use of hydrogenated and partially-hydrogenated oils. What is the reason? Could it have anything to do with the abundance of evidence screaming that hydrogenated oils interfere with normal cell function and are basically poison? Maybe you've heard of the alias "trans-fat."

So, what about food ingredient labels? As consumers we need to see through the savvy marketing buzz words like "all natural." So-called "all natural" products may still contain harmful ingredients.

Not to worry. Just make a habit of quickly reading ingredient labels. This can be a fun activity at the grocery store. Pretend you are an ingredient investigator on a mission.

Growing up, I knew nothing about ingredient labels. I probably ingested enough Yellow No. 5 to turn the color of the Sun. Now that I pay attention to the labels, seeing the ingredient "natural flavors" makes me curious enough to call the food manufacturer. It turns out that animal derived ingredients can exist within the "natural flavors" realm.

Avoid High-Fructose Corn Syrup–it's the United States' leading sweetener.[16] It tampers with blood sugar levels and is linked to obesity and diabetes.[17] Once you start reading ingredient labels, you'll find High-Fructose Corn Syrup everywhere. It's in breads, beer, soda, tonic water, cereals, ketchup, pasta sauces, and many other products. The average American consumes about 62 *pounds* per year![18] Food manufactures love to use it because it's cheap.

Consumers have begun to reach an *awareness* tipping point about the dangers of High-Fructose Corn Syrup. Now food companies will market the fact that they no longer use it. You've probably seen a product at the store with a standout blurb on the package that says something like, "now with no High-Fructose Corn Syrup."

It sounds nicer than saying, "we got away with selling you harmful ingredients for *years*, but since you found us out, we've changed our evil ways!" It's a good sign. That kind of *purchasing power* is proof that consumers are in command when they demand better products.

Aspartame is another deadly ingredient. You'll find this one in diet sodas, chewing gum, and any products that contain NutraSweet or Equal. The fact that the Food and Drug Administration allows Aspartame in our food reinforces that we shouldn't blindly trust what they say.

Aspartame consumption can include side effects like severe depression, anxiety, birth defects, headaches, migraines, nausea, bloating, and weight gain.[19] Yeah, you read it right. Diet sodas can actually keep people overweight! Can it get any more misleading?

There's an even darker story about this villainous Aspartame. One of the ingredients in Aspartame is methyl alcohol. When ingested, methyl alcohol converts into *formaldehyde*! Can you believe it? Formaldehyde is a known carcinogen and a deadly neurotoxin.[20] Formaldehyde, by definition, is "used in solution as a strong disinfectant and preservative."[21] Hmm. I wonder if it preserves fat cells too.

Phenylalanine is another concerning ingredient within Aspartame. When elevated levels of phenylalanine are present in the brain, serotonin levels in the brain decrease while the likelihood of depression, schizophrenia, and even seizures increases.[22] High levels of phenylalanine have been found in the brains of Aspartame consumers.[23]

When people purchase chewing gum, diet soda, or other products laced with Aspartame, it isn't their intention to be investing in suffering. Unfortunately, suffering is the long-term result. An awareness tipping point would help a lot of people.

Other artificial sweeteners to avoid include saccharin, acesulfame, cyclamates, neotame, and sucralose. Again, it all comes down to what's good for your body's pH.

Artificial sweeteners are all acidifying.[24] The ingredient label might as well spell out the word "p-l-a-g-u-e" instead of listing the artificial sweetener.

GREAT SWEETENER ALTERNATIVES

If you're looking for healthy sweetener alternative, try Stevia. It doesn't alter blood sugar levels.[25] It's also a non-caloric sweetener, available at larger grocery stores. Guess what? It's not artificial! Stevia is a herb native to Paraguay. Another natural sweetener option is agave nectar.

MSG GOES INCOGNITO

I thought I'd become a pro at spotting MSG, or Monosodium Glutamate, on ingredient labels. That all changed the day I watched a profound documentary film titled *The Beautiful Truth*.

Did you know that MSG can be within other ingredients on a label? It's quite a brilliant disguise. This means that restaurants can say they don't use MSG, maybe even with the best intentions, even though they are using MSG disguised under a different ingredient name.

Here some ingredient names where MSG can appear incognito: Monopotassium glutamate, Glutamate, Glutamic Acid, Gelatin, Hydrolyzed Vegetable Protein, Hydrolyzed Plant Protein, Autolyzed Plant Protein, Sodium Caseinate, Calcium Caseinate, Textured Protein, Yeast Extract, Yeast food or nutrient, and Autolyzed Yeast. [26]

Here's a brief explanation of why MSG is no good. It interferes with brain function and brain development. It is linked to diabetes and making cancer grow faster.[26]

Here's an exercise for shock value: google search MSG in infant formula. This is another example that shows how important it is to see through savvy marketing that does anything it can do to create the illusion of safety.

Here's a tip: if reading ingredient labels begins to be a chore, focus on eating the organic whole foods that are guaranteed MSG-free.

KEEP YOUR pH EYES OPEN

Just because a product donates proceeds to some cancer fund or heart disease organization doesn't mean it's helping you stay healthy. Keep your eyes peeled! There's always a marketing angle used to hook consumers.

Once you start paying attention to the pH of foods, you'll see right through the food and beverage manufacturers that are misleading consumers. Grocery store aisles offering meat and dairy products begin to look as if they are stocked with closure.

4) DAIRY IS A CON

"The human body has no more need for cows' milk than it does for dogs' milk, horses' milk, or giraffes' milk."
– *Michael Klaper, M.D., Author of "Vegan Nutrition: Pure & Simple"*

Discover more vegan tips & vegan recipes online at
www.StreetSmartVegan.com/blog

We've all heard the saying, "milk does a body good." Let's take a closer look to see if this is true. It's time to put an end to the shotgun spread of misinformation by the dairy industry once and for all.

Humans are the only animal species that consume milk after infancy. We're also the only species that consumes milk from other species! It walks the line of insanity because the nutritional requirements are very different for cows and people.

Too long has the dairy industry been misinforming. Especially advertising that drinking milk will give you strong bones. Guess what! We've been duped! It reminds me of the saying, "the bigger the lie, the easier it will be for people to believe."

OSTEOPOROSIS

Bone loss is *accelerated* by eating too much protein. Milk has such a high protein content, it's been called "liquid meat."[27] Humans simply do not need such a potent source of food. Why?

Dietary protein increases production of acid in the blood.[28] Remember, our blood has a pH balance that is slightly alkaline. Calcium is the alkaline shield that helps the body deal with too much protein. In order to balance out the increased acidity from excess protein intake, the body *leaches* calcium from the bones.[29]

Even though there is calcium in milk, the protein content is too high to make the equation work. The calcium is not "available." In the long-term, osteoporosis is the result. It's totally preventable.

ABSORBING CALCIUM

For the body to absorb calcium, it needs comparable amounts of magnesium.[30] The fact is, dairy products contain only small amounts of magnesium. Magnesium is the center atom of what I like to call "plant blood," or chlorophyll.[31] Green leafy vegetables contain a healthy balance of magnesium and calcium.[32]

Chlorophyll is the all-time essential. It alkalizes your pH level, purifies your blood, and helps blood cells transport oxygen all through the body. It also cleanses the liver and other organs from binding carcinogens.[33]

Fact: in 1931 Nobel laureate Dr. Otto Warburg proved that cancer cannot grow in a oxygen-rich environment. So, why not give your body a chlorophyll boost to get the oxygen moving?

I like to buy liquid chlorophyll and add it to filtered water. I do this at least twice a day. I have one friend that accuses me of "photosynthesizing" as I continue with my long-winded response about the benefits of chlorophyll.

DAIRY = SUFFERING

So what's the end result of consistently eating dairy? Dairy products like milk and cheese result in increased acidity for your body's pH.[34] Remember in the previous chapter about over-acidity being the root cause of all disease?[35] Well, keep in mind that cheese might taste great, but it's nothing more than highly concentrated milk.

Piles of scientific evidence say that dairy consumption carries disease baggage such as diabetes, constipation, ear infections, sinus congestion, rhinitis, rashes, dermatitis, eczema, hives, acne, asthma, digestive disturbance, irritable bowel syndrome, Crohn's disease, arthritis and joint pain, cancer (lymphoma, leukemia), obesity,[36] attention deficit disorder, heartburn, anemia,[37] heart disease, colic, allergies, autism, breast cancer, and prostate cancer.[38] Nothing tastes as good as vitality feels.

UNWANTED RESULTS OF INCREASED MILK PRODUCTION

Pesticides, antibiotics, hormones, and steroids are all found in dairy products.[39] Recombinant Bovine Growth Hormone, or rBGH, is a genetically engineered hormone that's injected into cows in the US. It was approved by the Food And Drug Administration in 1993 and *man* does it increase milk production! An increase in production of 10 to 15 percent. Why would all 25 nations of the European Union, Japan, Canada, Australia, and New Zealand decide to *ban* the use of the rBGH hormone?[40]

rBGH increases milk production by stimulating a cell growth hormone in cows called Insulin-Like Growth Factor-1. When humans drink this milk, we also ingest some Insulin-Like Growth Factor-1 and it makes our cells, *even cancer*, multiply faster. Humans don't need to be ingesting cell-growing hormones! Studies have connected the rBGH hormone with increased risk of colon, breast, prostate, lung, and pancreatic cancers.[41]

If that didn't alarm you, this might. Cows injected with Recombinant Bovine Growth Hormone are working overtime producing more milk than they normally would. Mastitis, an infection of the udders, increases dramatically. The infection is treated by dosing the cows up on antibiotics. The Centers for Disease Control warns that overuse of agricultural antibiotics is the largest promoter of food-borne, antibiotic-resistant infections in humans.[42]

Prepare yourself, because now it starts to get gross. When the cow udders are infected with mastitis, somatic pus cells form. There's actually an allowed amount of pus in milk! The Food and Drug Administration says that up to 750,000 somatic pus cells per milliliter of milk is acceptable.[43]

Synthetic steroids are also used to enhance milk production in the United States. Canada won't license the use of steroids because of evidence of increased cancer risk.[44] Irony arrives as baseball players in the U.S. get pressed in court for steroid use while the Food and Drug Administration approves the sale of milk contaminated with steroids.

I bet no celebrity would display their mug on a milk mustache advertisement if they knew that antibiotics, hormones, pus, and steroids end up in the milk supply. Every time I see a milk mustache billboard I think, "if they had just done *a little* research!"

DAIRY ALTERNATIVES

On the bright side, the United States *is* the largest market for dairy alternatives.[45] If you must have a milk-like or a cheese-like substitute in your diet, there's no shortage of tasty selections.

For milk alternatives, you can choose from almond milk, coconut milk, soy milk, hemp milk, rice milk, or even oat milk varieties. From the visual appeal of the product packaging to the way these options taste, none of these are as boring as milk from a cow.

When choosing, it all depends on what consistency you prefer. The nice thing is that if you want a break from one brand, variety is on your side. Above all, you know you'll be investing in a cholesterol-free beverage your taste buds will enjoy.

For cheese alternatives, one popular brand that won the VegNews product of the year award in 2009 is Daiya vegan cheese. Watch it melt at daiyafoods.com.

Here's a tip: for some alternative cheese products, the target market is vegetarian, not vegan. So when selecting a cheese substitute, make sure the ingredients don't list casein. Casein is the main protein present in milk.

5) MEAT IS DEAD ENERGY

"The beef industry has contributed to more American deaths than all the wars of this century, all natural disasters, and all automobile accidents combined. If beef is your idea of "real food for real people" you'd better live real close to a real good hospital."
– *Neal Barnard, M.D., Author of "Breaking the Food Seduction"*

Meat is dead. Dead with no beneficial enzymes. Meat has an acidic effect on the body that brings the pH level out of balance.[46] It's why people might sit on the couch for hours after eating animal for dinner while their body digests.

If you're looking for optimal energy, eating meat won't deliver. Why? A cow eats plant fibers that contain stored solar energy. A cow then converts the solar energy into flesh. You're getting secondary energy.[47] The cow beat you to it.

BIO-ACCUMULATING TOXINS

Bio-accumulation means that toxins will accumulate higher on the food chain. Animal products contain the toxins that are stored in animal's fat cells. The hormones, pesticides, antibiotics, and steroids found in animal products also magnify the acidic backlash on the consumer's pH.[48]

And, because "modern" meat production is so intensive, the fat content is up to *seven times* higher compared to non-industrialized meats.[49] This means more fat cells to store harmful toxins.

THE PROTEIN FRENZY...IS IT LEGITIMATE?

Of course the meat industry loves to turn attention away from how much harm animal products cause. Everyone's attention is fixed on protein. Protein has been the industry's most successful marketing diversion.

The number one question people ask me is: "If you are vegan, where do you get your protein?" People generally assume that protein doesn't exist beyond animal products! It's what they've been misled to believe.

Dr. Robert Young, in his book *The pH Miracle*, recommends 25 grams of protein per day. The average meat, dairy, and egg eating American most likely gets 75 to 125 grams per day![50] It becomes too much for the body to deal with.

In his book *The China Study*, Dr. T. Colin Campbell reveals, "The people who eat the most animal protein have the most heart disease, cancer, and diabetes."[51] His insight is based on over 25 years of research.

If you are worried about getting enough protein, forget it. If you eat a wide variety of vegetables, you are covered. Amino acids are the building blocks of protein, and vegetables have all the body needs.[52]

For example, the percentage of calories from protein in spinach is forty-nine percent. The percentage of calories from protein in iceberg lettuce is twenty-seven percent.[53]

IS TOO MUCH PROTEIN BAD?

What you should be concerned with is getting too much protein. Why? The body uses alkaline calcium from the bones to buffer the increase of acidity caused by excess protein consumption. Brittle bones, or osteoporosis, is the result.[54] So much for the protein frenzy.

Do animals that are much bigger and stronger than humans need to eat meat for proper protein intake? Nope. Elephants and horses get along just fine without it. What do they eat? Elephants eat a combination of leaves, twigs, grass, bark, seed pods, and fruit.[55]

YOU DON'T EVEN NEED ANY EXTRA CHOLESTEROL

The human body makes all the cholesterol it needs. This common knowledge is frequently forgotten. As

Dr. T. Colin Campbell explains in *The China Study*, "Lower blood cholesterol levels are linked to lower rates of heart disease, cancer, and other Western diseases."[56]

What makes cholesterol levels increase? Eating meat from animals. Animal foods are the only dietary source for cholesterol.

What makes cholesterol levels decrease? Dr. T. Colin Campbell's research explains, "nutrients from plant-based foods were associated with decreasing levels of blood cholesterol."[57]

Many times I've overheard people say, "high cholesterol levels run in the family." Listen, I'm not a guru nutritionist, but what would happen if everyone with high levels of cholesterol stopped eating animal products altogether?

MEAT ALTERNATIVES

Veggie burgers, tofu hotdogs, alternative deli slices, meat-less meatballs, and more. In fact, there's a substitute for any meat product you can think of. This means you can still enjoy some of your old favorite recipes!

Here's a tip: Try bringing tofu hotdogs or veggie burgers to that upcoming grill party. Everybody wins. The "grill master" will get introduced to the adapting times, your friends will have the opportunity to try something new, and you get to feast.

P.S. WANT MORE ENERGY?

Where can we locate the best sources of energy to supercharge the body's cells? Firsthand solar energy from uncooked vegetables, greens, and sprouts.[58] Foods that contain chlorophyll are supreme. Animal products and processed foods are prone to age and hinder our cells. Raw foods like wheatgrass restore vitality.[59]

Adding raw foods and wheatgrass to your diet will allow your cells to store a maximum electrical energy charge.[60] Ever feel the energy delivered from a shot of juiced wheatgrass? It's intoxicating.

Many cultures have become accustomed to heating foods. Clearly it's easier to digest some dense vegetables when they are steamed. Broccoli is a good steamer. But is it energy-efficient to always cook vegetables?

When vegetables are heated, beneficial enzymes are destroyed quickly. Cooking makes them nutritionally dead.[61] Consider the crunch of a raw green pepper. The vitality and crunchiness are lost when the green pepper is heated. With fresh and raw foods, you're guaranteed to get all the energy the food has to offer.

6) CLEAN WATER IS YOUR BUDDY

"I have from an early age abjured the use of meat, and the time will come when men such as I will look on the murder of animals as they now look on the murder of men."
– *Leonardo da Vinci*

Discover more vegan tips & vegan recipes online at
www.StreetSmartVegan.com/blog

Going to the grocery store with my 3-gallon jugs to stock up on reverse-osmosis filtered water is an enjoyable errand. Drinking cloudy tap water that tastes like a swimming pool...not so enjoyable. It's true, I'm a water snob, and I'll tell you why.

WATER BRINGS YOU VITALITY

Ready for a shocking statistic? 75% of Americans are chronically dehydrated.[62] This is perhaps the biggest cause of avoidable suffering. Ask yourself, "How many years have I been chronically dehydrated?" This is why hydrating needs to be a daily priority.

The human body is 70 percent water. The blood is 94 percent water.[63] It makes sense to provide the body with plenty of good water. Hydrating with pure water is not to be confused with drinking beverages that *contain* water. The coffees, teas, sodas, or energy drinks won't cut it. None of these are as effective in hydrating the body as plain water.[64]

Dr. F. Batmanghelidj, in his book *Your Body's Many Cries For Water*, has done noteworthy work that everyone should know about. The main talking points include, "It is chronic water shortage in the body that causes most of the diseases of the human body" and "you are not sick, you are thirsty."[65] You can look into these points further if you visit watercure.com.

YOUR BODY WILL LET YOU KNOW

Dr. Batmanghelidj writes that a "dry mouth" is not the only indicator of body thirst.[66] Asthma, allergies, unexplainable chronic pains, arthritis, heartburn, and headaches might also be translated as thirst signals.[67] Dark colored urine is also an indicator of dehydration.[68]

How much water should you drink in a day? That answer is relative to many factors, but a *minimum* of six to eight 8-ounce glasses of water is what the body needs.[69]

In February of 2005, I learned this lesson the hard way. I experienced what Dr. Batmanghelidj calls "False Appendicitis Pain."[70] I knew Appendicitis was common in our family. So, when the mysterious pain in my lower abdominal region persisted for days, I became concerned enough to go to the emergency room.

They found no evidence of Appendicitis and sent me home. It was a confusing evening. What was the problem? I wanted answers.

Weeks later, after reading *Your Body's Many Cries For Water*, it became clear that I was chronically dehydrated. My body was just trying to tell me. I didn't understand the thirst feedback signal.

Now I drink nearly a gallon of water a day. To alkalize water, squeeze in lemon or lime. Adding liquid chlorophyll also alkalizes water. Mint flavored liquid chlorophyll added to water is especially refreshing.

When drinking water, it's important to sip instead of guzzle. Think about a soaker hose in a garden. It allows plants to absorb water slowly instead of drenching them all at once. Sipping water throughout the day allows the body a proper chance to absorb.

SALT IS ESSENTIAL

Proper hydration cannot occur without salt intake. Salt allows our cells to retain water. Dr. Batmanghelidj recommends adding a half a teaspoon to the diet for every 10 glasses (two quarts) of water.[71]

Are all types of salts the same? No. Most table salts are bleached to look white and some have unwanted additives to enhance taste. You'll want to look for unrefined sea salt. Even better, check out Redmond RealSalt.

Redmond RealSalt is harvested near south central Utah where an ancient sea once existed. Volcanos erupted, sealing in layers of salt deposits that remain unpolluted to this day.

Zinc, Copper, Manganese, Iodine, Phosphorus, Iron, Magnesium, Sulphur, Potassium, and Calcium are all beneficial trace minerals found in Redmond RealSalt. It tastes way better than common table salt too.

THE GRIM TALE OF TAP WATER

If you drink *tap* water, it might be keeping you alive, but it's not helping you thrive. From what I've observed, many people believe that tap water isn't harmful because it's tested and approved.

But, safety isn't a requisite of approval. There are enough contaminants in tap water for an entire book to be written on the subject. To keep things simple, we'll just focus on two commonly known tap water additives.

Let's start with the poison called chlorine.[72] Chlorine isn't the most advantageous means of disinfecting our water, but it sure is the cheapest![73] Chlorine might be cheap to put in the water, but what is the price in suffering for people who drink it?

The U.S. Council Of Environmental Quality says, "Cancer risk among people drinking chlorinated water is 93% higher than among those whose water does not contain chlorine."[74] Why? Chlorine in water is carcinogenic, it promotes free radicals that cause cell damage.[75]

Let's move on to the next poison in tap water, fluoride.[76] We've been told for years that it's good for our teeth. There's only one problem, it isn't true![77] It's been proven that fluoridation does not reduce tooth decay.[78]

Fluoride is nothing more than an industrial waste product and a known carcinogen.[79] Ninety percent of the fluoride added to tap water consists of hydrofluoric acid which is a chemical compound of fluoride.[80] Fluorine is a chemical by-product of various manufacturing industries.[81] So why is fluoride, an active toxin in rat poisons,[82] added to drinking water at low levels?

Mostly because it provides manufacturing companies a profitable means of disposing of their industrial waste. Although, fluorides are also effective in modifying the mood and behavior of human beings.[83,84]

One not widely talked about bit of history is that fluoride compounds were added to the drinking water in Nazi prison camps in order to keep prisoners submissive and to discourage the questioning of authority.[85] Apathy, anyone?

CONSISTENT POISON IN SMALL AMOUNTS

It's important to think about the *long-term* consequences of consistently ingesting a poisonous substance, even if it's in small proportions. While writing this chapter on water I received the 2008 Water Quality Report in the mail for the city I was living in, Grand Rapids Michigan. It was in this city that the environmental hazard fluoride was first added to tap water around 1945.

The report lists the highest level of fluoride detected at 0.95 parts per million.[86] The report also lists that fluoride is a "water additive which promotes strong teeth."[87] This is simply not true.

Studies have shown that drinking water with fluoride at units of 1 part per million can have alarming consequences. It may look like a low amount on paper, but fluoride concentrations at 1 part per million speed up the aging process and increase the release of harmful free radicals in the body. It also weakens the immune system by interfering with the movement of white blood cells to infected locations.[88]

Keep in mind, 1 part per million is merely .05 units *above* the 0.95 parts per million of fluoride that the Environmental Protection Agency considers safe for my city. A difference of only 5 percent.[89] Does that mean it's safe?

No. Consuming fluoride in water is not safe. I don't even like using it in toothpaste. It's a classic example of people being misinformed, then using something without doing their own research. Kind of like the idea of mercury tooth fillings!

When I went to the dentist as a child, they required me to swish a fluoride solution in my mouth for at least a minute, it may have been longer. That stuff tasted like it didn't belong anywhere *near* my mouth.

Here's a tip: if you're looking for awesome toothpaste that's natural and organic, try the JASON brand. Their fluoride free "Power Smile" variety is incredible. You're likely to find this brand at your local health food store.

GETTING CLEAN WATER

There are many water filtration products out there. Although, if you are going to invest in one for long-term use, do plenty of research. Some products talk a big game yet don't deliver where it counts. For example, a Brita filter has it's limitations.

My suggestion is to get reverse-osmosis filtered water from the grocery store. Many grocery stores have these filter stations in the water aisle. It costs about twenty-nine or thirty-nine cents per gallon. From what I've researched, it's a beneficial and cost-effective solution. Your body will thank you.

7) INTERVIEW WITH A VEGAN MOTHER

The following interview is with the person who first introduced me to the benefits of being vegan. Her vegan wisdom has prompted what I like to think of as my life's most adventurous detour. She is a humble encyclopedia of health and nutrition information.

What truly makes her an authority on all matters vegan is that she doesn't just know the information, she's lived it. Her knowledge is derived from the most solid source: *experience*.

Jay Wesley Anderson – **JWA**:

Lilian, thanks for agreeing to do this interview. You're the mom in a vegan family with a 4-year-old vegan child. It's not exactly following the crowd when it comes to diet choices for raising a family. ***What made you choose a vegan diet?***

Lilian Bernal Anderson – **LBA**:

Becoming vegan was an evolution from being vegetarian, and prior to that, I was like most folks, living by the standard "pyramid diet" recommended by the American Nutrition charts…drink your milk for calcium, eat your meat for protein, etc.

More than a diet, vegan is a way of life; it's a lifestyle! It all started by listening to the signs from my physical health…allergies, poor digestion, insomnia, etc. After growing up in Colombia, where the water, air, and the overall goods produced by the local agriculture, are clean and "untreated" compared to the U.S. standards, I realized that most of my health challenges were mostly related to my diet. My mother always told me so! (It took me a while to listen). When I moved from Colombia to the U.S. I was sick all the time. It was part physical and part emotional. A poor diet did not help the overall picture.

Part of my "dietary evolution" was thanks to the influence of my mother, she pioneered an alternative lifestyle within the traditional walls of our family's circle. She was vegetarian, practiced yoga and meditation, used natural remedies whenever possible, all this when it was not popular or mainstream as it is today. She studied macrobiotics, integrative nutrition and has been working in the field of alternative medicine and detoxification of the body since I was a kid. So the inspiration to look at other avenues was always there, thanks to her role model.

I never enjoyed eating animal derived foods, so becoming vegetarian was easy. What was truly life changing was becoming vegan. Vegan not only includes what we eat, but also the choices we make in the clothing we wear, the personal care items we use and the entertainment we choose. I believe, and know with my heart and soul that in this lifetime, animals are not ours to eat, wear, experiment with or use as entertainment. So, becoming vegan was seeing the world and my role in it from a completely different perspective from how I was raised to believe.

I think, and without judging others, that

"living" and choosing a compassionate lifestyle, will give me and my son, a better chance to create a happier, healthier life on this planet for all. And as humans, I hope to leave a lighter footprint. The earth needs it, we all need it to thrive, not just survive!

As a mother, it's a blessing that my husband is also vegan. He wasn't before we met, but as he slowly incorporated foods that were lighter, greener and vegetarian, he noticed healthy changes in his body. And as more information came his way, it was an easy transition. Again, he did it by free will, it's the only way to create change, through freedom of choice without too much preaching! (Haha).

JWA: In the United States we are blitzed by advertisements from the dairy industry. Many parents are misled to think that their kids won't grow properly if they don't drink cow's milk. ***Has the vegan diet you've chosen interfered with your child's growth rate in any way?***

LBA: No. Not at all! On the contrary, my beautiful four-year-old son has thrived with good health and normal mental, physical and emotional development. I am grateful for his good genes. Most of all, I'm grateful for the choices we've made since he was conceived. Keep in mind that a healthy mama will most likely have a healthy pregnancy, delivery, and thus, a healthy child.

I had an awesome pregnancy (never sick) and felt amazing. The delivery was the same, just wonderful, and although I encountered some individual challenges related to postpartum (due to stress, lack of rest, etc). I can't imagine how things would have been if we had a different diet and lifestyle!

I also think that mother's milk makes a tremendous difference in kids. If a mother can nurse, she should give it a try. It's not easy, but it's a gift to ourselves and to our children! It builds their immune system and nourishes the child in so many wonderful ways. For a mother it is a precious and unique time with her baby.

Our son has had the normal incidence of colds like any other child that attends nursery school (part time) and let me tell you, it's less than the average. He is building his immune system with the unavoidable viruses from other kids. However, his overall health is remarkable–and now I'm quoting the pediatricians that have checked him since birth! His recovery time from any virus is fast compared to other kids.

In fact, he had a massive ear infection in both ears. We decided against surgery. That not only could have impaired his hearing for life, but he could have also faced the risk of brain damage! The little guy fought it and flushed the infection with the guidance and help of our pediatrician, our Acupuncture Chinese M.D., and unfortunately, a round of strong antibiotics. And even after all the sleepless nights and medications, he bounced back to full strength in record time!

At the pediatricians office and at the ear, nose, and throat specialist's practice, his ears are still mentioned "as a remarkable case of recovery without surgery." I am grateful for the vegan diet and lifestyle. I know that helped.

And regarding his growth and general physical strength, it is normal and his mental development is very advanced for his age. And this is not just a mention from his bragging parents, it's what teachers and pediatricians have told us too.

I do know that a vegan diet has kept at bay all the terrible diseases related to sugar, milk, and all the artificial stuff that kids have these days as the norm. For example, diabetes, asthma, skin eczemas, re-occurring ear infections, obesity, sleeping, and behavioral disorders, etc. It's awful. So many kids just in nursery school and already at the hands of pharmaceutical remedies (drug dependency) due to terrible health issues. Very sad and all due to lack of information.

JWA: We've talked before about the importance of positive affirmations the expression of gratitude to promote well-being. Films like The Secret and What the Bleep Do We Know are inspiring testimonials of the power our thoughts can have. *Are there any affirmations that you use when you cook that you'd like to share with those reading?*

LBA: I love this question! Yes, I do try to be present and mindful when prepping meals. In my native country, Colombia, peasants that worked at our house as cooks or housekeepers, would always say, "Never cook with a hot head or a sobbing heart… it ruins the flavor!"

And since our son was born, I am particularly careful about that. I remember when I was nursing him, I would look at my milk and think of how it would nourish him, how much love he was receiving and how it would make him strong. I continue to do this when I cook for my son or husband.

I think of love, calming feelings and comfort. In such a rushed and busy world, the thought of receiving this kind of positive energy through a meal is healing. I believe in the healing (or destructive) power of thoughts. It's extraordinary what the mind can do to the body!

Stress is a state of mind that kills slowly. The body is just a manifestation of mental and emotional pollution. Children are radars for this kind of energy. Their spirits and minds are so light and clear that they can quickly become hosts for all kinds of negative vibes.

Eating should be a mindful, calming moment. A time to break from everything and nourish. And in today's world, sadly, that's just something we do on special occasions. That's why I dislike and avoid eating and watching TV or movies with negative, heavy content. Talk about indigestion!

TACO RECIPE FROM A VEGAN MOM

The Vegan Taco Mix:

1. Tomato base stock/soup half cup (more or less–depending on how dry or moist you like your mix).
   Note: My favorite tomato stock/soup brand, always in my pantry: Imagine Foods Organic Creamy Tomato Soup (Vegan).
2. Chopped/well-diced ripe tomatoes, two medium or one big one.
3. Chopped scallions, these are the long green onions (one stalk or more depending on size) or one-half red onion/diced.
   Note: scallions are milder, red onions are a bit more bold/flavorful.
4. Bell pepper, one-half of a big green or red bell pepper, chopped well.

To your palate's taste:
Organic Ground Cumin
Organic Garlic Powder
Organic Chili Powder
Organic Sea Salt

Optional:

If you like spicy foods (hot) add organic cayenne powder

Step 1- Mix all the above ingredients in a medium heated pan and sauté until the tomatoes, onions and peppers are tender and well mixed with the tomato stock.

Step 2- Mix in (2 packs) Yves Meatless/Ground Taco Mix Original (Vegan) (I prefer the original because you can add more or less condiments to taste). Mix and blend the taco mix with your sauce until all is well sautéed in to a thick mix, not watery or runny. Taste to check. Add salt/spice, etc.

Step 3- Add to mix: Fresh cilantro (a small bunch) coarsely chopped. Mix in well without overcooking to add color and flavor. Turn heat off. Let mix stand/cool off.

Step 4- (Optional) Avocado add-on for your taco:
One(1)or two(2)fresh crushed organic ripe avocados.
Fresh organic lemon or lime juice (to taste).
Sea salt (to taste).
Minced scallions and cilantro to taste.
Mix all the above.

Set on a dish/bowl to serve on the side or add/layer last to your taco.

Build Your Vegan Taco

Ingredients:
1. Taco Shells/Wraps
2. Organic Corn (Vegan) Taco Shells (the toasted kind) My favorite brand: Bearitos Organic Yellow Corn Taco Shells

Optional:
Soft Vegan-Organic White Wraps, Yellow Corn Wraps, Whole Wheat Wraps, or Soft Sprouted Grain Wraps, Fresh organic green lettuce or collard greens used as a wrap.

Step 1- In your taco shell or wrap, place one or two lettuce leaves.

Step 2- Add two or three tablespoons of the sautéed taco mix.

Step 3- Layer the avocado mix (optional) or serve on the side.

Step 4- Garnish with more cilantro to your taste (optional).

Buy organic ingredients as your first choice always! Enjoy![90]

QUICK LINKS TO RECIPE PRODUCTS

1. yvesveggie.com/products/detail.php/meatless-ground-round-original
2. wholefoodsmarket.com/products/item.php?RID=147
3. littlebearfoods.com/products/index.php

8) ADRENALINE, NOT FOR CONSUMPTION!

"If slaughterhouses had glass walls, everyone would be a vegetarian."
– *Paul McCartney*

When a person eats meat, not only are they getting a ton of cholesterol they don't need, they're also eating adrenaline![91] Adrenaline in meat exists as a result of the methods used during the slaughtering process.

Animals, like you and me, are intelligent, emotional, and social creatures.[92] Animals get afraid when they sense danger. To ready themselves for the terrifying event of slaughtering, animals release high amounts of adrenaline that remain in meat until it's on the dinner table. Adrenaline is highly toxic in this form. Meat eaters ingest this toxicity.[93]

Would it surprise you to learn that beef products labeled as "free-range" aren't strictly regulated by the United States Department of Agriculture?[94] It's mostly a marketing ploy to make people feel better about buying. When it comes to the slaughtering, it's pretty much all the same. It's far from quick and painless.[95]

NOT SO NICE

While researching, I stumbled upon many disgusting practices happening at factory farms. Details so graphic they were difficult to finish reading. If you want to know more about what's happening to animals at factory farms, you can visit peta.org.

I've read about cows, pigs, chickens, and turkeys basically being tortured alive in the worst way during the slaughtering process.[96] Living conditions while animals are *alive* are cramped.[97] It's understandable why a lot of people are sincerely upset about animal cruelty and won't eat meat for that reason alone.

Surely it depends on how seriously you want to think about what you're eating and where the energy has come from. Could it be that people are ingesting the funky energy from any suffering occurred in an animals life? I personally have a hard time not thinking about food that way. Yet another reason why vegetables are so light and enjoyable.

EYE TO EYE

Picture early winter driving through Wisconsin, dairy capital of the U.S. I was on the highway passing a truck loaded with cows. Through the open-air gate in the side of the truck I glanced over at a cow. It gave me a long look in the eye. At that time I was in the beginning stages of this book. It was a defining moment.

HOW TO GIVE AWAY A LEATHER COAT

"The love for all living creatures is the most noble attribute of man."
– *Charles Darwin*

Step 1: Be grateful for the time you spent with the coat. It kept you warm. It made you look cool. It made you feel like you looked cool.

In order to complete step 1, you must put your coat on one last time and have a reflection moment. Focus on the gratitude you feel for the coat and the animal that made the coat possible. Appreciate the time you had with the coat. Ahh... now you have a nice thing called closure.

Step 2: Know that it will keep someone else warm. Know that it will make someone else look and feel cool. The animal that died so this coat could exist did not die in vain. The coat will be put to more good use.

Step 3: Know that the coat will benefit someone else at a fair price. How? Because you are going to give the coat to a charity store that will resell it. You can then feel even better knowing that the charity place will earn money on the re-sale and put that money toward doing more good.

Step 4: Make the give. Feel good about making the give. It's a good give. Wait! Don't forget to check all coat pockets. And if you really want to make someone's day, leave a $1 bill on purpose.

10) HUMAN ANATOMY TELLS NO LIE

"If humans were carnivores, we'd be sweating through our tongues instead of our skin." [98]
– *Dr. Robert O. Young,*
Author of "The pH Miracle"

It's taken millions of years of evolution to create the human body we now experience. Carnivores and herbivores have prominent anatomy differences. Let's see what distinctions reveal the most conclusive evidence.

DIGESTION

To aid in digestion, carnivores have stomach acid concentrations that are about 10 times that of humans and herbivores.[99] The stomach size of a carnivore, such as a lion, is about 65 percent of the entire capacity of the digestive system. Their main goal is to quickly swallow as much meat as possible and then rest to digest.[100]

Herbivores and humans have a more complex digestion process. It begins in the mouth. We need to chew our food before swallowing it. Unlike carnivores, our saliva contains the enzyme Alpha-Amylase. This enzyme allows us to digest plant foods and carbohydrates.[101, 102]

TOOLS OF THE TRADE

Carnivores have canines and claws to tear flesh. Humans need to use tools like the fork and knife. Human evolution has gifted humans with an opposable thumb that allows for efficient gathering of foods with a high content of water and fiber.[103]

THE INTESTINES OF A CARNIVORE

Meat contains no fiber. Once digested, meat decomposes faster than vegetables. Evolution has effectively equipped carnivores with intestines as short as 3 times the length of their body. The decomposing meat doesn't have much intestinal space to linger before it passes out of a carnivore's body.[104]

YOU'VE GOT A LOT OF GUTS

Herbivores and humans have intestines that are 10 to 12 times their body length.[105] Our anatomy favors spending a longer time digesting foods that are high in water content and decompose slowly.[106] Vegetables fit the part.

Human intestines are too long to support a high meat diet. The dead meat simply has too much space to sit, rot, and cause problems.[107] Just because humans can eat meat, doesn't mean it's efficient for our insides.

FIBER IS YOUR FRIEND

Fiber is the glue that attaches to harmful carcinogens to transport them out of the body.[108] Because animal products are loaded with fat and cholesterol, they cause an increase in bile-acid production to help with digestion. Once this bile-acid gets to the colon, it is converted into carcinogens by the colonic bacteria. The risk of developing colon cancer increases the more animal products a person eats.[109] Fortunately, fiber helps prevent the intestines from absorbing cholesterol.[110]

Trouble arrives for people who eat meat as a staple part of their diet because they most likely aren't getting enough fiber. The daily average of fiber intake for Americans is between 10 and 15 grams.[111] This is especially alarming in the U.S. where the population consumes high fat meats like beef for 40% of their total fat calorie intake.[112]

In the United States, products that advertise "a good source of fiber" practically leap off the shelf. It's become a wonderful selling point. A large population of meat eaters have become increasingly aware fiber's benefits. They just haven't been told to cut out the root source of the problem.

If you are eating a plant-based diet, you have no problem getting enough fiber. Eating 35 grams of fiber per day is recommended.[113] That might seem like a lot. It isn't once you start replacing meat with other staple plant-based foods.

11) BEST THING YOU CAN DO FOR THE PLANET

"Nothing will benefit human health and increase chances for survival of life on Earth as much as the evolution to a vegetarian diet."
– *Albert Einstein*

Discover more vegan tips & vegan recipes online at
www.StreetSmartVegan.com/blog

GLOBAL WARMING: WHAT IS IT?

Have you ever noticed that the term "global warming" has been branded so that most of the attention is directed toward the emissions from cars, factories, and the industrial revolution?
You might be amazed to discover this, but where it counts the most, a vegan diet works like magic to lessen the amount greenhouse gases emitted by humans.

Greenhouse gases are exactly what they sound like, they trap warmth inside the atmosphere of the Earth. Just like windows in a greenhouse. To a point, greenhouse gases are a good thing, actually they keep our planet warm enough to live on!

The truth is, we humans are holding on to some seriously inefficient cultural practices. You know, I'm talking about eating animals!
As you will discover below, if humans don't curb their appetite for flesh and animal products, the warming will continue and start causing consequences not ideal for our own survival.

NUMBERS SPEAK LOUDER THAN WORDS

Being vegan is *by far* the best thing each of us can do to alleviate environmental stress from the planet. That's a fact. Seventy percent of all agricultural land on Earth is used for livestock production. This figure combines grazing area and land dedicated to feed-crop production. Guess what? That's 30 percent of the planet's *entire* land surface! All dedicated to livestock production![114]

Seventy percent of once forested land in the Amazon is occupied by pastures.[115] Not only has the lush bio-diversity suffered, trees that help balance the carbon cycle have been taken out of the equation.

A PLANET IN NEED OF EFFICIENCY

The planet can feed more people subsiding on a plant-based diet. On the amount of land it takes to feed one person with an animal-based diet, we could be feeding about 17 people on a plant-based diet.[116] What could a massive shift toward veganism do for world hunger?

Consider that it takes 4.8 pounds of grain to make one pound of beef. Producing one hamburger patty uses the equivalent of enough fuel to drive 20 miles.[117] The livestock industry uses far more energy than it yields!

In the United States, animal production uses more than a third of all fossil fuels and raw materials.[118] Think energy savings. Think pollution prevention.

THE BIG PICTURE

Whether you want to call it global warming or climate change, it's happening. The livestock sector is *the most overlooked* source of the problem. Get ready, you're about to learn the most overwhelming fact that is changing global warming conversations around the world!

Here is the dirty little secret the livestock sector doesn't want you to know:

18 percent of greenhouse gas emissions measured in carbon dioxide equivalent come from the livestock sector. This is a higher percentage than transport.[119]

THE WRATH OF THE LIVESTOCK SECTOR

Guess what one of the biggest polluters is...it's shit! Manure and wastewater containing manure from factory farms messes up river and stream ecosystems. It's a problem because manure contains ammonia *highly* toxic to fish at low levels.[120]

A 2006 report published by the United Nations Food and Agriculture Organization gets more specific. They found that livestock are responsible for 64 percent of all ammonia emissions. Acid rain and the acidification of ecosystems is the result.[121] There's more. Increased amounts of the nutrients nitrogen and phosphorus that flow into waterways from animal feeding operations cause algal blooms. These algal blooms heist oxygen from waterways in order to decompose.[122]

In 1996, factory farms in the U.S. created 1.4 billion tons of animal waste. The Environmental Protection Agency has reported that animal waste pollutes American waterways more than all other industrial pollution sources combined.[123]

Livestock industries are responsible for over 8 percent of global human water use. Watering feed crops is largely what creates this percentage.[124] Does it make sense to allot a significant percentage of the water supply to livestock industries? They have an end game that massively pollutes our overall water supply!

POPULATION GROWTH

Ever had the thought that there's too many people on the planet? In 2005, there were about 20 billion head of livestock on Earth. Roughly triple the number of people![125]

The United Nations estimates that global population is expected to reach 9.1 billion by the year 2050.[126] If a large portion of the population still subsides on a heavy meat diet, can you imagine the stress it will cause to the environment? Being vegan is like giving an advance gift to help in sustaining the environmental future of the planet.

EACH PERSON'S ECOLOGICAL "FOOTPRINT"

Unless you've been living under a rock, you've heard about greenhouse gasses. They enhance global warming. Your lifestyle choices determine how much your unique eco-footprint affects the global environment. Are you stepping lightly or are you stomping?

A 2005 University of Chicago study showed that even a vegetarian who still eats dairy is responsible for much less greenhouse gas emissions than someone consuming a standard meat-rich American diet. The difference equals roughly 1.5

metric tons of carbon dioxide per year when calorie intake is equal.[127]

In other words, becoming a vegetarian has the same affect on carbon dioxide emissions as the difference between driving a Chevrolet Suburban and a Toyota Camry.[128] A vegan footprint is less.

Going vegan would reduce the greenhouse gas emissions discharged from producing what you eat more than seven-fold![129] This is the kind of efficiency makes me feel excited, empowered, and optimistic about the environmental future of this planet.

What else can you do to make your ecological footprint lighter? Support local growers and embrace simple, organic, non-genetically modified living. Does it make sense to buy a vegetable or a bottle of water that was shipped from hundreds or even thousands of miles away? Those products may be cheap, but what is the *hidden* price that environment is paying to get those products produced and then transported the distance?

HOW TO BE SURE YOU'RE BUYING ORGANIC

Look at the sticker on the produce. The organic produce SKU number begins with 9, as in #90442. The conventional produce SKU number begins with the number 4, as in #4554. Also, organic produce is always marked. If it's unmarked, it's conventionally grown.

WHY IS ORGANIC PRODUCE BETTER?

Buying genetically modified crops is basically voting for the increased use of polluting chemicals.[130] Plus, how can we possibly know the ripple effect that genetically engineered plants will have? It's basically introducing new D.N.A. combinations in to the environment, toying with evolution. Why not simplify the equation and eat organically grown foods?

Many people think organic foods are too expensive. Actually, organic vegetables are more nutritious than non-organic vegetables, with up to 40 percent more antioxidants.[131] By eating organic foods, you are investing in a higher quality of life... and that is priceless.

HOW MUCH HAS EARTH ACTUALLY WARMED UP?

NASA did a study in 2006 revealing that the Earth has been warming approximately 0.2 degrees Celsius (.36

Fahrenheit) each decade for the last 30 years.[132]

Some might say, "that seems like a small number of degrees of warming, why should that be alarming?" For starters, the survival of plant and animal species is dependent on established temperature ranges.

Even though the warming in recent decades seems slight when you read it on paper, it is causing animals in the Northern Hemisphere to migrate toward the North Pole.[133]

That almost sounds too crazy to be true, but it is! A 2003 study showed that 1700 insect, plant, and animal species have moved poleward at an average rate of 4 miles each decade in the last half of the 20th century.[134]

12) CALL TO ACTION

> "It is my view that the vegetarian manner of living by its purely physical effect on the human temperament would most beneficially influence the lot of mankind."
> – *Albert Einstein, letter to Vegetarian Watch-Tower, 27 December 1930*

Discover more vegan tips & vegan recipes online at
www.StreetSmartVegan.com/blog

It's time to rally. If we want a secure homeland for future generations, it starts with the health of people and our surrounding environment. There's a large inventory of reasons why consuming animal products is not to our advantage as a species looking for long term survival.

The Environmental Protection Agency, Food and Drug Administration, and United States Department of Agriculture have yet to say "no" to giant corporations with large lobbying budgets. I don't think we should wait around for them to make change.

EMPOWERING SOLUTIONS

Ok, enough of the whining protest. Change will come from consumers. The responsibility is ours and ours alone. This is a much more empowering way to arrive at a solution. Guaranteed.

Our vote for a brighter future resides with the daily consumption choices we make. Remember, with our purchasing power, we create the demand which ultimately controls what kinds of products companies will supply. The change we need will continue as people get more informed about how their food choices affect themselves and the planet.

13) A VEGAN DAY

> "Whenever anyone asks me if being vegan means eating 'rabbit food,' I ask them if they've noticed how fast rabbits are."
> – Jay Wesley Anderson

For me, I know that being vegan allows me to function far more efficiently than the food choices I used to cling to. "You are what you eat" is a truism. It all comes down to the quality of fuel you are feeding your body.

I've met vegetarians with health problems, even overweight vegans. Puzzled at first, I realized that many people don't pay attention to pH and proper hydration as a street smart vegan would.

Many fad diets have people counting every little calorie. That's unrealistic. If you're eating foods that are keeping your pH alkaline, you don't need to waste your mind-power feeling guilty about eating too many calories. Give yourself a break!

HOW TO USE THIS CHAPTER

Try out some of the food ideas in this chapter and see if they work for you. Pay attention to the feedback your body is giving you. As you start to gauge how you feel from eating mostly alkaline foods, you will begin to understand how important pH really is. If you'd like to share what you think about any of the food options in this chapter, I'm listening. Email me: CustomerCare@StreetSmartVegan.com.

Even though this chapter focuses on food, it's always a good time to hydrate between meals. Remember, 6 to 8 eight-ounce glasses per day at minimum.

GOOD MORNING

Boot coffee. Kick it as far away from you as possible! The energy you get from coffee makes you the jittery captain of a sinking ship. You float for awhile and then you plunge into the energy abyss.

Coffee is street-stupid! Savvy marketing touts coffee's antioxidant content to boost consumer confidence, yet it crushes your pH. It is an acidic start to what could be a truly energetic, alkaline morning.

Try beginning your day with a glass of pure, room temperature water accompanied by some light stretching. Remember, sipping instead of guzzling will allow your body time to absorb. I prefer room temperature water instead of chilled or iced. Our 98.6 degree body has to expend energy to make a cold drink warm. After about 15 minutes, I prepare the following drink.

FEEL THE ENERGY FROM THIS TASTY GREEN SHAKE

In a blender or 16-ounce glass, stir the following ingredients:

6 to 8 ounces of pure water
4 ounces of original flavored rice milk
1 scoop of "green drink" powder
    (cleanses vital organs, alkalizes)
1 tablespoon or so of liquid chlorophyll,
    (purifies blood, helps oxygenate the body, deodorizes)
    Mint-flavored chlorophyll can also be used
1 tablespoon of flax seed oil
    (Essential omega 3, 6, & 9 fatty acids, promotes whole body well-being)
    Hemp seed oil can also be used for these benefits
1 tablespoon of pure soy lecithin granules
    (supports brain and nerve function and energy production)
2 ounces of aloe vera juice or gel
    (supports digestion, organ and tissue function)

HOW TO LOCATE THESE INGREDIENTS

I recommend going to your nearest health food store. Ask them about the "green drink" powders they offer. There are several brands to choose from. Once you've decided on your green drink powder, the soy lecithin granules, flax seed oil, aloe vera gel, and liquid chlorophyll should be easy to find.

WHY THE "GREEN DRINK" IS AWESOME

The green drink is an alkaline investment. It's quality energy. It's crash-free energy. It will help you maintain consistent well-being.

It's taking the concept of a multi-vitamin, changing up the ingredients, and putting it into and easily digestible liquid form. The best part about a green drink is drinking a second one later in the day if you want to.

Remember, this can be a gradual transformation. You might want to try adjusting to this green shake twice a week to start and then increase intervals in the following weeks. You may want to give your body time to adjust to absorbing these high-quality foods.

Imagine — a non-jittery morning, sitting with your green drink. You're celebrating the fact that you're no longer investing in your own acidic demise by drinking coffee every morning! Cheers!

So, what about making smoothies? Your blender has been missing you. Add the same green drink ingredients previously listed. This time add a tablespoon of any or all of the following options: goji berries, raw chocolate nibs, ground flax seed, or almond meal.

To give the smoothie a creamy consistency, try using a fresh (still a little green) banana. You may need to add a little water if it gets too thick. A handful of blueberries or a half gram of Stevia powder will deliver extra sweetness if desired.

BREAKFAST

It's time to look at breakfast in a new way. The breakfast foods you once invested in were probably wreaking havoc on your pH. I'm talking about the eggs, bacon, bagels and cream cheese, milk, cereal laced with High-Fructose Corn Syrup, and orange juice spiked with sugar.

LUNCH IS THE NEW BREAKFAST

I know…you're sick of hearing people say that this is the new that. Me too. This time it's true though! It's never too early in the day to eat foods that are alive with energy. That's right, vegetables! Here are a few options to start your day.

TASTY WRAPS

Wraps are great because they are a perfect way to visualize the 80:20 alkalizing ratio we talked about in Chapter 3. The grain-based wrap is the 20 percent acidifying portion and the vegetables loaded inside are the 80 percent alkalizing portion.

Remember at the end of Chapter 5 when we covered the electrifying energy delivered from raw foods? Well, wraps allow you to eat a bunch of raw vegetables in a convenient way, even at 7 in the morning!

A good brand for the wrap is the Food For Life brand's Ezekiel 4:9® Sprouted Whole Grain Flourless Tortilla. Begin the wrap by spreading on hummus. This helps hold together the vegetables and greens you add. Next, add a broad leaf of romaine lettuce. Then pile on the chopped vegetables.

Try any combination of the following: onions, green peppers, tomatoes, avocado slices, mushrooms, or sliced radish. Toss on some spinach. If you like herbs, be generous with adding chopped mint, cilantro, basil, or parsley. Drizzle some Annie's Goddess salad dressing. Cover all that with another broad leaf of romaine lettuce to help keep it together.

REMEMBER THE DAILY LARGE SALAD

Try a simple combination of spinach, romaine lettuce, sprouts, and chopped parsley, cilantro, basil, or mint. What if you want a more filling salad? Dice a small tomato and 7 ounces (1/2 a brick) of tofu.

Looking for a tasty salad dressing? Annie's Naturals Goddess Dressing will tempt your taste buds. The Annie's Naturals brand also has other vegan dressings, like Green Garlic.

WHY TO USE A GENEROUS AMOUNT OF HERBS

We all know that herbs deliver that extra touch of "wow" to any meal, but what makes them superior to stored spices? The fresh factor, and they are alkaline. On any meal, especially salads, try using generous amounts of mint, parsley, cilantro, or basil.

Buying herbs all the time isn't necessary. Herbs are extremely easy to grow. You don't even need a huge garden space.

HAVING LUNCH IN A HURRY? TAKE THIS SANDWICH WITH YOU

Remember in Chapter 3 how yeast products were on the list of acid forming foods? A healthy alternative to breads made from yeast and bleached flour is Ezekiel 4:9® Organic Sprouted Whole Grain Bread. It's made by a company called Foods For Life. If it's not on the shelves, look in the freezer section at your local grocery store.

So what goes between the bread? Spread on some hummus. Layer in some greens. Add in sliced red pepper, avocado, tomato, cucumber, onion, or any other alkalizing vegetable you like. Cut it in half so you can see your work of art!

ANYTIME, TAKE-ALONG SNACKS

The combination of raw chocolate nibs and goji berries is scrumptious. These are two of the most antioxidant-potent foods on the planet! This snack tops my list of staples to keep nearby.

Want an energy dense standby? Raw almonds are where the alkaline action is. Because almonds are alkaline, they are superior to peanuts. Soaking almonds in a bowl of water for an hour will make them plump and hydrated. They'll be easier to chew and digest. Almonds are a good source of vitamin E and magnesium.

Avocado is another alkaline champ. After cutting an avocado in half and removing the pit, two bowl-like spaces will remain. I like to add fresh salsa or tabouli, then spoon up the goodness.

Hummus is another healthy food to keep around. Celery, radish, cucumber, tomato, carrot, green peppers and zucchini are all good alkalizing vegetables to dip in hummus. Dashing on Redmond RealSalt to the sliced vegetables will enhance the taste.

THE HOME-MADE, MONEY-SAVING HUMMUS RECIPE

1. Soak 2 cups of chick peas in water for 24 hours to sprout.
2. Boil the chick peas and drain them once they are cooked.
3. Sqeeze the juice from 2 lemons.
4. Add 1 large clove of chopped garlic.
5. Add 1 teaspoon of unrefined sea salt.
6. Add 1/4 teaspoon of ground black pepper.
7. Add 1/3 cup of sesame tahini.
8. Add about 1 cup of water while blending to get the creamy consistency.
9. Blend all the above in a food processor...enjoy!

ENJOY LOW-SUGAR FRUITS

You might be wondering why I don't write much about fruit. Fruit is high in sugar. Sugar makes your pH acidic. There are great low-sugar fruits that have an alkaline effect on the body. Avocado, tomato, lemon, lime, and grapefruit fall into this category.

It's easy to eat a lot of watermelon, it's relatively low in sugar. Compare that to a fruit like pineapple which is so high in sugar that it becomes difficult for your taste buds to handle after awhile. Vegetables don't crash your pH and they give you all the nutritional benefits that high-sugar fruits can.[135]

I've experimented eating multiple servings of fruit, soy yogurt, and soy chocolate milk all in the same day. The result is always noticeable breakouts on my forehead. It's amazing how the body gives feedback. The lesson here is to consume fruit and other sugary foods in moderation.

DON'T FEEL LIKE COOKING?

Many grocery stores offer vegetable sushi made with brown rice. Look for rolls that include avocado, cucumber, or carrot.

Here's a tip: use Bragg's Liquid Aminos instead soy sauce. The taste is very similar and the Bragg's is certified Non-GMO. It also contains 16 beneficial amino acids.

Another tip: save the cap from a spent Bragg's Liquid Aminos container and use it for your liquid chlorophyll bottle. It makes it easier to dispense the chlorophyll.

AFTERNOON ALKALIZING

At some point in the afternoon, a wheatgrass drink always seems to be the answer. Pure Planet makes a product called Green Kamut. Add a teaspoon of this powder to 6 ounces of water and you've got supreme energy in a glass. It's a great ally for anyone on the go because it doesn't call for refrigeration. You get 90 servings for under $25. That's a cost-effective $0.27 drink.

THE DINNER OF A MULTI-TASKER

A rice cooker is a handy appliance. You can multitask while rice is cooking. Heat up some Organic Creamy Tomato Soup from the Imagine brand. When your brown rice is done cooking, you can add part of a container of Imagine soup on top.

To make the soup a bit more robust, add chick peas, soy, or navy beans. Add a tablespoon of olive oil and a pinch of Redmond RealSalt to taste. Set the rice cooker to warm, or turn it off. Simple.

While your rice cooks, chop up some broccoli and a garlic clove. Add about a cup of water to the bottom of a pot, toss in the broccoli and garlic. Cover and let it steam.

Then, chop up a sweet potato into cubes. Toss them into boiling water. When those are done, drain the water and add some Earth Balance Natural Buttery Spread. Add a pinch of Redmond RealSalt, several crushed cilantro seeds, a little dash of cayenne pepper powder, and garlic powder to taste. Mash it up if you want. If the consistency is too dry, add a little water.

So, you've been stirring soup, checking on steaming broccoli, and cooking sweet potatoes. Pretty soon you will sit down to a very satisfying meal. Warm meals always make the stomach feel content. Feel free to add freshly chopped cilantro, parsley, or basil!

BEING VEGAN & GETTING VITAMIN B-12

Vitamin B-12 is one supplement that any vegan should consider taking. Vitamin B-12 supports normal nerve and brain function.

I recently started to take a once or twice a week approach with a certified vegan B-12 supplement. The non-daily approach makes a ton of sense to me. Honestly, what is my body possibly going to do with a 50,000% Daily Value pill of B-12 everyday?

Along with taking a B-12 supplement a couple times a week, you can get B-12 in fortified vegan products like imitation meat and milk substitutes.

The importance of vitamin B-12 for vegans is a topic you might find mixed information about. For example, I've found research that says vegans don't need to worry about getting B-12 at all, that it is just another nutrition myth similar to what we've all seen with the "eat meat for protein" frenzy.

But I've also discovered that doctors recommend vegans take a B-12 supplement because it can't be acquired unless you eat animal products.

Here's a tip: it comes down to the peace of mind question, "Isn't it worth it to know that I'm covered on vitamin B-12 so I can ensure I will have normal brain and nerve function?" Absolutely.

WHAT HAPPENS IF YOU FALL OFF THE VEGAN BUS?

If you fall off the vegan bus, don't beat yourself up about it. Remember, if you're new to the vegan lifestyle, change requires flexibility. Be flexible with yourself. Pick up where you left off, and continue. Thinking too much about it can create unhealthy stress and anxiety.

Do I ever tumble off the vegan bus? It happens. I'm a survivor, and I don't like to think too strictly in absolutes. Besides, sometimes options are limited.

During your vegan transformation, you might find that your taste buds and food cravings change over time. For example, I no longer have an appetite for meat. But avoiding cheese can be tough sometimes. My body gives me mild digestion feedback reminding me that long-term, being vegan is the smartest choice to make. I jump back on the bus before it leaves me behind.

14)

3 COMMON MISTAKES NEW VEGANS MAKE AND HOW YOU CAN AVOID THEM

"To my mind, the life of a lamb is no less precious than that of a human being. I should be unwilling to take the life of a lamb for the sake of the human body."
– *Mahatma Gandhi*

COMMON MISTAKE #1:
OVER-EXTENDING A "LAZY VEGAN" PHASE.

The word is out. It is easy to be a lazy vegan...very enjoyable too! On the couch with a super quick dinner, no chopping necessary.

Let's face it, at the grocery store, the vegan goodies section is always looking better and better! You know...the meatless meatballs, vegan burger patties, or vegan ice creams.

Here's the important concept: it's ok to be really efficient at playing the role of the "lazy vegan," but for limited times only.

Frozen vegan foods are important to have around to supplement your vegan bag of tricks, but our bodies do well eating mostly uncooked fresh foods from the earth.

I'm talking about foods like avocados, leafy greens, and almonds.

Why? Raw foods are still "alive" with electrical energy. If you're ever feeling tired and run down, consider that you need to recharge.

So, what are some quality fuels that will help you recharge? Salads with plenty of leafy greens are always a good start.

If your lifestyle is on the go, try bringing along slices of cucumber, carrot, radish, or celery to dip in hummus.

COMMON MISTAKE #2: SPENDING TIME IN A VEGAN "BUBBLE."

Sure, it's easy to feel outnumbered as a vegan. But there's no need to let it reinvent your social life.

Actually, I've found that social outings surrounding food are more interesting as a vegan. Why? There's much more to observe and talk about.

Here's the important concept: to make social outings surrounding food enjoyable, all you have to do is satisfy people's curiosity!

Share a few healthy tips from your vegan bag of tricks. Let them in on a few tips or products to use that make eating vegan easy.

For example, you might mention that on sandwiches, there are some great mayonnaise substitutes available that work just as well.

Another example, on wraps, you can mention that replacing meat with avocado or hummus works great.

COMMON MISTAKE #3: NOT MEETING NEW VEGAN FRIENDS.

Maybe you've heard the saying, "You are who you hang out with." Let's examine why this is true.

If you're hanging out around fellow vegans, you'll probably be sharing tips, checking out healthy vegan additions on local restaurant menus, and giving positive encouragement when somebody falls off the vegan bus.

Here's the important concept: Hanging out with fellow vegans will reinforce your new lifestyle of choice.

To break the ice with your existing circle of friends, invite them over for some tasty vegan food.

If you don't get any takers, search online for a "vegan group" or "vegan meetup." These groups meet about once a month at restaurants that cater to vegan appetites just like yours.

15)

VEGAN ROAD-TRIPS: HOW TO TRAVEL HEALTHY AND COST EFFECTIVE

I have no doubt that it is a part of the destiny of the human race, in its gradual improvement, to leave off eating animals..."
– *Henry David Thoreau*

Discover more vegan tips & vegan recipes online at
www.StreetSmartVegan.com/blog

People drive cars. Most cars run on gas. People that sell gas figured out quickly that they could only locate filling stations no more than a certain number of miles apart, or else cars would run out.

Fast food chains adopted a similar strategy by default. It goes like this: when people stop for gas, they can also stop for food so quickly and easily…that they don't even have to get out of their cars to get fed!

The only problem is…fast food sucks. It's horrible for you. It costs you money but it makes you feel crappy.

Ok — maybe Subway has a veggie sub with no cheese that can get you by in pinch if they absolutely load on the spinach. Then add whatever veggies you like…tomato, onion, green pepper, olives, lettuce. And condiments…mustard or spicy mustard, or olive oil. If Subway had hummus, that would really be something. The good news is that Subway's Italian bread has no animal derived ingredients.

So what is the solution? How can you make your vegan road trip healthy and cost effective?

If you look at it from a cost: benefit viewpoint, stopping at the local grocery stores that are just a short distance, if not across the street from the fueling station is much healthier and cost effective.

Suddenly, an entourage of recipe of options open up. You can now buy food that gives you the real energy you are looking for. These are some of the same easy vegan recipes you've already learned in this book.

What do you toss in your shopping basket? Purchase ingredients to make easy vegan wraps, sandwiches, and even greens to make salads.

Just make sure you bring a few essentials such as a cooler, a cutting board that doubles as a serving plate, a bowl for salads, and necessary tools to eat with…fork, spoon etc. Wraps and sandwiches are easy to eat on the road.

Locate a loaf of vegan bread or a packet of wraps, then spread on hummus, layer on spinach and/or romaine lettuce, then layer on any of the following: sliced tomato, avocado, sliced red pepper, sliced firm tofu, or alfalfa sprouts.

Have questions or comments? Please contact us at
CustomerCare@StreetSmartVegan.com

16) SOCIAL OUTINGS SURROUNDING FOOD

"We must be the change we wish to see in the world."
– *Mahatma Ghandi*

I'm grateful that both of my siblings are vegan, so family meals are no sweat. Having a support network of like-minded people works wonders to positively reinforce any lifestyle of choice.

If you're interested in dining with people on a similar vegan wavelength, try searching "vegan groups" online and join one in your town. The vegan meetup in my town bounces around to various restaurants once a month. I've also heard of vegan retreats that include lodging and vegan meals lasting for up to a month.

GOING OUT TO EAT

Going out to eat with non-vegan friends or business associates is no big deal. You don't have to choose a special restaurant that makes the evening revolve around your unique diet, just be prepared to entertain people's curiosity.

It's human nature for people to be afraid of what they don't understand. Don't be offended if people throw the outcast vibe at you. And don't feel like you are offending if someone asks you, "What's so bad about what I eat?" Tell it like it is–because it is.

ORDERING A DRINK

After you've been a street smart vegan for a few months, paying attention to pH will be second nature. You'll be able to quickly scan past the sugary, carbonated sodas laced with caffeine. Those drinks have "pH inefficiency" written all over them.

If you're used to drinking purified water, it's easy to tell if water at a restaurant is any good. I usually take my chances and order a glass of water with no ice. I ask for lemon or lime slices to make the beverage alkaline. Since I hydrate between meals, I don't normally drink that much water while eating.

ORDERING A MEAL

When ordering meals I've found that restaurants are usually happy to entertain vegan requests. Menus usually list salads, soups, and appetizers that work fine. When a salad has meat in it, ask them to leave it out or replace it with avocado or tofu.

If you can't locate a vegan dish on the menu, ask for non-dairy or no meat preparation. It's a simple request. At the very least, you'll be giving feedback to the restaurant that their menu needs some reinventing.

YOU JUST BLEW YOUR COVER!

Now that you've ordered your meal and voiced your seemingly unique food preferences, curiosity is in the air. All eyes on you! Good thing you know your stuff, right?

PREPARE TO ANSWER THESE QUESTIONS

Someone is sure to ask you, "What made you decide to go vegan? To keep the answer short, yet informative, it helps to stick to two basic talking points. Try responding, "I enjoy the health benefits and I feel good about leaving a lighter environmental footprint."

Remember, the people you are dining with have probably been fed misinformation for most of their lives. They are comfortable clinging to the idea they've known for years that animal products are beneficial.

People resist change. They might not want to get what you are saying. If they agree with you, they'll have to admit that they've been duped their entire life by the clever marketing of meat and dairy companies.

SPEAKING ON BEHALF OF THE VEGAN LIFESTYLE

When people ask you questions, think of it as a unique opportunity to speak on behalf of the vegan lifestyle. It's important! So if one of your talking points is "health benefits," be prepared to expand on that.

What health benefit is most worth mentioning? Everyone will appreciate hearing about how vegan foods are naturally cholesterol free.

You might also mention a few of the avoidable dis-eases that come from consuming animal products. These were covered in Chapters 4 and 5.

Or talk about how much more energy you have now that you stay away from foods like meat and dairy that crash your pH.

Be ready to answer this question too…"Why is a vegan diet more environmentally friendly?" In Chapter 11, you'll find some percentages that will hook interest.

Try mentioning, "70 percent of all agricultural land on Earth is used for livestock production."[136] People understand percentages easily.

Here's a tip: concrete facts satisfy curiosity and boost your credibility as a speaker. Use them to your advantage.

EASY TABLE CONVERSATION TRANSITIONING

When the above conversation starts to burn out, you could rattle off a few of those household names mentioned in Chapter 1 who corroborate your story. Who knows, the conversation might push forward to global warming and the entire dinner party might consider adopting a vegan lifestyle.

You'll be surprised at how receptive people are when they hear a few grounded talking points. So make sure you ground your talking points!

FINAL REMARKS

By now you've learned some information that will add to your quality of life. If you have questions, email me: CustomerCare@StreetSmartVegan.com. Now I'll say farewell.

5
BONUS VEGAN RECIPES

Discover more vegan tips & vegan recipes online at
www.StreetSmartVegan.com/blog

A LAZY VEGAN BREAKFAST

- Heat oven to 450 degrees
- Place 2 frozen Hash Brown Potato Patties on a baking sheet (find them in the frozen aisle near hash browns)
- Cook in oven. After 6 minutes, flip potato patties
- Cook for 6 more minutes, then remove baking sheet from oven
- Lightly spread Vegenaise (Follow Your Heart brand) over potato patties
- Layer salsa or pico de gallo over potato patties to taste
- Optional: combine with steamed broccoli

TRAVELING SANDWICHES

- Lay out 4 slices of Ezekiel 4:9 Sprouted Grain Bread
- Spread hummus over all 4 bread slices
- Add 2 ounces of alfalfa sprouts to each sandwich
- Add a broad leaf of romaine lettuce to each sandwich
- Drizzle on a tablespoon of Annie's Goddess Salad Dressing
- Top it off with a layer of spinach
- Add top bread slices and press down to compact the sandwiches for travel
- Slice as needed to fit your travel container
- Sandwiches are cleared for takeoff

FRESH & ENERGIZING SALAD

According to Dr. Robert O. Young, Director of Research at the pH Miracle Living Center, "eating alkaline fruit and vegetables is the best way to build healthy blood and a strong, healthy body."

In a large bowl, add the following:
- one generous handful of spinach
- one chopped head of romaine lettuce
- 2 sliced radishes
- One cubed avocado
- one half cup of cubed tomato
- Dressing Option: Annie's Goddess Salad Dressing
- Mix and enjoy!

THE REVIVE WRAP

- Lay out 3 broad romaine lettuce leaves side by side on a cutting board
- Layer on hummus lightly
- Overlap the middle edges of the lettuce leaves by 1 inch, using the hummus as the "glue" that will hold wrap sections together. Now you should have 3 connected lettuce leaves laying flat.
- Add a handful of living mung bean sprouts
- Add slices of red, yellow, orange, or green pepper (use 1/3 of a pepper total)

- Add a generous amount of fresh parsley or cilantro to taste.
- Fold the wrap together, make the hummus work like the seal of an envelope

BERRIES ON A BOAT

- Lay out three sticks of celery on a plate
- Spread Almond Butter in the grooves of the celery sticks
- Sprinkle Goji Berries on top of the Almond Butter

About This Recipe:

The Berries On A Boat Recipe was heisted from the 'ants on a log' snack concept. Remember that one? Celery, peanut butter, and raisins posing as ants. The upgrade needed to be made for the following reasons:

Eating raisins can get boring. Offering berries cruising on a boat at 50 m.p.h. can light up a room!

The better health reasons for the recipe upgrade:
Almond Butter is by far a higher quality food than the peanut butter called for in the 'ants on a log' snack. Why? Because almonds are alkaline.

What's story with the goji berry? Why are they so great to have in your entourage? For starters, the goji berry is one of the most nutrient-rich foods on earth.

Goji berries enhance immune system function and circulation. They are also a solid source of antioxidants.[137]

Sources Consulted

"24 Potentially Harmful Food Additives." Accessed April 14, 2009, wereyouwondering.com/possible-and-suspected-carcinogens-found-in-food/

"Animal Waste: What's the Problem?" Environmental Protection Agency. Accessed December 30, 2009. epa.gov/region09/animalwaste/problem.html

Aronson, Dina., M.S. R.D. "Vegan Nutrition with Dina Aronson, M.S. R.D." VegFamily. Accessed March 11, 2009. http://www.vegfamily.com/dietician/0804a.htm

"Aspartame Side Effects." Dr. Janet Hull. Accessed March 14, 2009. sweetpoison.com/aspartame-side-effects.html

Barnouin, Kim, and Freedman, Rory. Skinny Bitch. Philadelphia: Running Press Book Publishers, 2005.

Batmanghelidj, F., M.D., Your Body's Many Cries For Water. Vienna: Global Health Solutions, Inc.,1997.

Bigmore, Susan. "Soy Good For You." July, 2003. Accessed April 14, 2009. functionalingredientsmag.com/fimag/article Display.asp?strArticleId=68&strSite=FFNSite

Breyer, Mellissa. "Cow Milk: Easy Greening."
April 17, 2006. Accessed April 15, 2009. care2.com/
greenliving/cow-milk-easy-greening.html#

Butler, Graham., BCS., CNPA. "The Truth
About Milk." Alive, April, 2003: 72-74.
enzymeuniversity.com/artman/publish/
article_20.shtml

Campbell, T. Colin., Ph.D., and Campbell,
Thomas. The China Study: Startling Implications
For Diet, Weight Loss And Long-Term Health. Dallas:
BenBella Books Inc., 2006.

Castel, Vincent. et al., Livestock's Long Shadow:
Environmental Issues and Options. Food and
Agriculture Organization Of The United Nations. 2006.

"Chlorine, Cancer, And Heart Disease." Global Healing
Center. Accessed April 23, 2009.
ghchealth.com/chlorine-cancer-and-heart-disease.html
City of Grand Rapids Water System. Water
Quality Report. 2008.

Cohen, Robert. "MILK A-Z," Accessed January 14,
2009, http://www.notmilk.com.

Cox, Jeff. "The Organic Food Shopper's Guide." New
Jersey: Wiley & Sons Inc. 2008.

Davis, Gail. "A Tale of Two Sweeteners: Aspartame & Stevia," accessed April 12, 2009, suewidemark.netfirms.com/davis.htm

"Elephant." African Wildlife Foundation. Accessed April 18, 2009. awf.org/content/wildlife/detail/elephant

"Famous Vegetarians." Accessed December 30, 2008. vegetarian-restaurants.net/OtherInfo/FamousVeg.htm.

"Fiber-Recomendations" Accessed May 26, 2010. umm.edu/ency/article/002470rec.htm

"Fluoridated and Chlorinated Water: Wide Range of Serious Health Problems." Shirley's Wellness Cafe. Accessed April 23, 2009. shirleys-wellness-cafe.com/fluoride.htm

"Fluoridation. Mind Control of the Masses." Stephen, Ian E., The Truth Campaign. Accessed April 23, 2009. ivanfraser.com/articles/health/fluoride.html#top

"Formaldehyde" Def. 1. Webster's New World College Dictionary. 3rd ed. 1997

Fox, Dr. Michael W., Eating With A Conscience. The Bioethics of Food. Troutdale: NewSage Press, 1997.

"Free-Range Eggs and Meat: Conning Consumers?" Peta.org. Accessed April 28, 2009.
peta.org/mc/factsheet_display.asp?ID=96

Gold, Mark D. "The Bitter Truth about Artificial Sweeteners." truthcampaign.ukf.net. Accessed April 13, 2009, truthcampaign.ukf.net/articles/health/aspartame.html

Goldhamer, Alan, D.C. "No Body Needs Milk: 10 Reasons For Avoiding Dairy Products," Accessed January 14, 2009.
vegsource.com/articles2/goldhammer_milk.htm

"Healthiest Diet Ever." Posted November 20, 2007. Accessed April 15, 2009. veganjacks.blogspot.com/

"Here Are 10 Physical Differences Between Carnivores (Meat Eaters) And Herbivores (Plant Eaters). Is The Human Body Designed To Eat Animal Products?" Accessed April 14, 2009. http://www.waoy.org/26.html

Howard, Brian C. et al., Green Living: The E Magazine Handbook For Living Lightly on the Earth. New York: Penguin Group, 2005; 4, 9, 15.

"Jupiter Melody Water Ionizer." Accessed April 23, 2009. phmiracleliving.com/p-175-jupiter-melody-water-ionizer.aspx

Koerner, Brendan I., "Vegans vs. Vegetarians, What Kind of Diet is Best for the Environment?" Slate, October 23, 2007. Accessed December 30, 2008, slate.com/id/2176420/

"Milk Sucks." Peta.org; milksucks.com. Accessed January 17, 2009. milksucks.com/

Mills, Milton R., M.D. "The Comparitive Anatomy of Eating." Accessed January 14, 2009. http://www.vegsource.com/veg_faq/comparative.htm

"More about Raw Chocolate Benefits." Accessed April 17, 2009. chocchick.com/more-about-raw-chocolate-benefits-913-0.html

"NASA Study Finds World Warmth Edging Ancient Levels." http://www.nasa.gov/vision/earth/environment/world_warmth.html

"Scientific Facts on the Biological Effects of Fluorides." Natural Health and Longevity Resource Center. Accessed April 23, 2009. all-natural.com/fleffect.html

Shiva, Vandana. Stolen Harvest: The Hijacking Of The Global Food Supply. Cambridge: South End Press, 2000.

Simone, Charles B. M.D., Cancer and Nutrition. A Ten-Point Plan to Reduce Your Risk of Getting Cancer. New York: Avery Publishing Group Inc. 1992.

"Soft Drinks, High-Fructose Corn Syrup Promote Diabetes, Says Study." March 10, 2005. Accessed April 14, 2009, naturalnews.com/002584.html

The Beautiful Truth. Cinema Libre Distribution. 2008

"The Hidden Lives of Chickens." Peta.org.
Accessed April 27, 2009.
peta.org/feat/hiddenlives/

"The Toxic Effects of Fluoride." Wholy Water.
Accessed April 23, 2009.
wholywater.com/fluoride.html

"The Vegan Facts." Total Raw Food. Accessed April 27, 2009. totalrawfood.com/rawfood/&cat=20&p=25

"Tibetan Goji Berries." Accessed April 17, 2009.
tibetgojiberry.com/

"Tiny Vegan Footprints" Gluten-Free Vegan.
September 2, 2008. Accessed June 15, 2009.
glutenfreevegan.wordpress.com/2008/09/02/146/

Vasey, Christopher. N.D., The Water Prescription. For Health, Vitality, and Rejuvenation. Vermont: Healing Arts Press, 2002.

Wagen, Stephen N.D. "Food Allergy Solutions Review. News, Ideas & Strategies to Improve Your Health." July 2003. Accessed January 15, 2009. foodallergysolutions.com/food-allergy-news0307.html

"Why Be A Vegan / Vegetarian?" February 17, 2003. Accessed March 24, 2009.
stephen-knapp.com/why_be_a_vegan_vegetarian.htm

"Why Vegetarian?" Accessed December 30, 2008. archure.net/salus/vegetarian.html Wigmore, Ann. The Wheatgrass Book. New Jersey; Avery Publishing Group Inc, 1985.

Wong, Cathy. What Are Goji Berries? August 1, 2006. Accessed February 14, 2010. http://altmedicine.about.com/od/completeazindex/a/goji.htm

"World Population To Increase By 2.6 Billion Over Next 45 Years." Press Release POP/918. United Nations. February 24, 2005. Accessed March 14, 2009. un.org/News/Press/docs/2005/pop918.doc.htm

Young, Robert O., Ph.D., and Shelley Redford Young. The pH Miracle: Balance Your Diet, Reclaim Your Health. New York: Warner, 2002.

Endnotes

1) Koerner., "Vegans vs. Vegetarians - What kind of diet is best for the environment?" slate.com/id/2176420/

2) "Famous Vegetarians" vegetarian-restaurants.net/OtherInfo/FamousVeg.htm

3) "Healthiest Diet Ever," veganjacks.blogspot.com/

4) Young., 7.

5) Young., 5.

6) Young., 6.

7) Young., 51.

8) Young., 51.

9) "More about Raw Chocolate Benefits," chocchick.com/more-about-raw-chocolate-benefits-913-0.html

10) "More about Raw Chocolate Benefits," chocchick.com/more-about-raw-chocolate-benefits-913-0.html

11) "More about Raw Chocolate Benefits," chocchick.com/more-about-raw-chocolate-benefits-913-0.html

12) "More about Raw Chocolate Benefits," chocchick.com/more-about-raw-chocolate-benefits-913-0.html

13) "Tibetan Goji Berries," http://www.tibetgojiberry.com/

14) "Tibetan Goji Berries," http://www.tibetgojiberry.com/

15) "Tibetan Goji Berries," http://www.tibetgojiberry.com/

16) Howard, et al., 9.

17) "Soft Drinks, High-Fructose Corn Syrup Promote Diabetes, Says Study," naturalnews.com/002584.html

18) Howard, et al., 9.

19) "Aspartame Side Effects." sweetpoison.com/aspartame-side-effects.html

20) Young., 89-90.

21) "Formaldehyde" Def. 1. Webster's New World College Dictionary, 530.

22) Gold, "The Bitter Truth about Artificial Sweeteners," truthcampaign.ukf.net

23) "24 Potentially Harmful Food Additives," wereyouwondering.com/possible-and-suspected-carcinogens-found-in-food/

24) Young., 89

25) Davis, "A Tale of Two Sweeteners: Aspartame & Stevia," suewidemark.netfirms.com

26) The Beautiful Truth. Cinema Libre Distribution. 2008

27) Cohen, "MILK A-Z," notmilk.com

28) Cohen, "MILK A-Z," notmilk.com

29) Young., 78.

30) Cohen, "MILK A-Z," notmilk.com

31) Cohen, "MILK A-Z," notmilk.com

32) Young., 78.

33) Young., 52.

34) Young., 51.

35) Young., 6.

36) Goldhamer, "No Body Needs Milk: 10 Reasons For Avoiding Dairy Products," vegsource.com/articles2/goldhammer_milk.htm

37) Wagen, "Food Allergy Solutions Review." foodallergysolutions.com/food-allergy-news0307.html

38) "Milk Sucks," milksucks.com

39) Barnouin., 60.

40) Breyer, "Cow Milk: Easy Greening." care2.com/greenliving/cow-milk-easy-greening.html#

41) Breyer, "Cow Milk: Easy Greening." care2.com/greenliving/cow-milk-easy-greening.html#

42) Breyer, "Cow Milk: Easy Greening." care2.com/greenliving/cow-milk-easy-greening.html#

43) Breyer, "Cow Milk: Easy Greening." care2.com/greenliving/cow-milk-easy-greening.html#

44) Butler, "The Truth About Milk." enzymeuniversity.com/artman/publish/article_20.shtml

45) Bigmore, "Soy Good For You." functionalingredientsmag.com/fimag/article Display.asp?strArticleId=68&strSite=FFNSite

46) Young., 51.

47) Wigmore., 11.

48) Young., 81.

49) Shiva., 66.

50) Young., 84.

51) Campbell., 102.

52) Young., 61.

53) Young., 62

54) Young., 78-79.

55) "Elephant," awf.org/content/wildlife/detail/elephant

56) Campbell., 78.

57) Campbell., 80.

58) Wigmore., 11.

59) Wigmore., 4.

60) Wigmore., 2.

61) Howard, et al., 15.

62) "Jupiter Melody Water Ionizer." phmiracleliving.com/p-175-jupiter-melody-water-ionizer.aspx

63) Young., 92.

64) Vasey., 1.

65) Batmanghelidj., xvii.

66) Batmanghelidj., 9, 21.

67) Batmanghelidj., 21, 35, 41, 51.

68) Batmanghelidj., 158.

69) Batmanghelidj., 151.

70) Batmanghelidj., 35.

71) Batmanghelidj., 161.

72) Young., 93.

73) "Chlorine, Cancer, And Heart Disease." ghchealth.com/chlorine-cancer-and-heart-disease.html

74) "Chlorine, Cancer, And Heart Disease."
ghchealth.com/chlorine-cancer-and-heart-disease.html

75) "Chlorine, Cancer, And Heart Disease."
ghchealth.com/chlorine-cancer-and-heart-disease.html

76) Young., 93.

77) "Fluoridated and Chlorinated Water: Wide Range of Serious Health Problems."
shirleys-wellness-cafe.com/fluoride.htm

78) "The Toxic Effects of Fluoride."
wholywater.com/fluoride.html

79) "Fluoridated and Chlorinated Water: Wide Range of Serious Health Problems."
shirleys-wellness-cafe.com/fluoride.htm

80) "Fluoridated and Chlorinated Water: Wide Range of Serious Health Problems."
shirleys-wellness-cafe.com/fluoride.htm

81) "Fluoridated and Chlorinated Water: Wide Range of Serious Health Problems."
shirleys-wellness-cafe.com/fluoride.htm

82) "Fluoridated and Chlorinated Water: Wide Range of Serious Health Problems."

shirleys-wellness-cafe.com/fluoride.htm

83) "Scientific Facts on the Biological Effects of Fluorides."all-natural.com/fleffect.html

84) "Fluoridation. Mind Control of the Masses." ivanfraser.com/articles/health/fluoride.html#top

85) "Scientific Facts on the Biological Effects of Fluorides." all-natural.com/fleffect.html

86) City of Grand Rapids Water System. Water Quality Report. 2008.

87) City of Grand Rapids Water System. Water Quality Report. 2008.

88) "The Toxic Effects of Fluoride." wholywater.com/fluoride.html

89) City of Grand Rapids Water System. Water Quality Report. 2008.

90) Anderson, Jay. Interview with Lilian Bernal Anderson. 14 June. 2009.

91) "The Vegan Facts." totalrawfood.com/rawfood/&cat=20&p=25

92) "The Hidden Lives of Chickens," Peta.org

93) "The Vegan Facts." totalrawfood.com/rawfood/&cat=20&p=25

94) "Free-Range Eggs and Meat: Conning Consumers?" Peta.org

95) Barnouin., 77.

96) Barnouin., 77.

97) Fox., 26.

98) Young., 83.

99) "Here Are 10 Physical Differences Between Carnivores (Meat Eaters) And Herbivores (Plant Eaters). Is The Human Body Designed To Eat Animal Products?" http://www.waoy.org/26.html

100) Mills., "The Comparitive Anatomy of Eating." http://www.vegsource.com/veg_faq/comparative.htm

101) "Why Be A Vegan / Vegetarian?" stephen-knapp.com/why_be_a_vegan_vegetarian.htm

102) Mills., "The Comparitive Anatomy of Eating." http://www.vegsource.com/veg_faq/comparative.htm

103) "Here Are 10 Physical Differences Between Carnivores (Meat Eaters) And Herbivores (Plant Eaters). Is The Human Body Designed To Eat Animal Products?"
http://www.waoy.org/26.html

104) "Why Be A Vegan / Vegetarian?"
stephen-knapp.com/why_be_a_vegan_vegetarian.htm

105) "Why Be A Vegan / Vegetarian?"
stephen-knapp.com/why_be_a_vegan_vegetarian.htm

106) "Here Are 10 Physical Differences Between Carnivores (Meat Eaters) And Herbivores (Plant Eaters). Is The Human Body Designed To Eat Animal Products?"
http://www.waoy.org/26.html

107) "Here Are 10 Physical Differences Between Carnivores (Meat Eaters) And Herbivores (Plant Eaters). Is The Human Body Designed To Eat Animal Products?"
http://www.waoy.org/26.html

108) Simone., 235.

109) Simone., 231, 234, 235.

110) "Vegan Nutrition with Dina Aronson, M.S.R.D." http://www.vegfamily.com/dietician/0804a.htm

111) "Fiber-Recomendations" umm.edu/ency/article/002470rec.htm

112) Simone., 233.

113) "Fiber-Recomendations" umm.edu/ency/article/002470rec.htm

114) Castel, et al., xxi.

115) Castel, et al., xxi.

116) "Why Vegetarian?" archure.net/salus/vegetarian.html

117) Howard, et al., 4.

118) Howard, et al., 4.

119) Castel, et al., xxi.

120) "Animal Waste: What's the Problem?" epa.gov/region09/animalwaste/problem.html

121) Castel, et al., xxi.

122) "Animal Waste: What's the Problem?"
epa.gov/region09/animalwaste/problem.html

123) Howard, et al., 4.

124) Castel, et al., xxii.

125) Howard, et al., 4.

126) "World Population To Increase By
2.6 Billion Over Next 45 Years."
un.org/News/Press/docs/2005/pop918.doc.htm

127) Koerner., "Vegans vs. Vegetarians - What
kind of diet is best for the environment?"
slate.com/id/2176420/

128) Koerner., "Vegans vs. Vegetarians - What
kind of diet is best for the environment?"
slate.com/id/2176420/

129) "Tiny Vegan Footprints." glutenfreevegan.
wordpress.com/2008/09/02/146/

130) Shiva., 101.

131) Cox., 27.

132) "NASA Study Finds World Warmth Edging
Ancient Levels." September 25, 2006.
Accessed December 31, 2009.

http://www.nasa.gov/vision/earth/
environment/world_warmth.html

133) "NASA Study Finds World Warmth Edging Ancient Levels." September 25, 2006. Accessed December 31, 2009.
http://www.nasa.gov/vision/earth/
environment/world_warmth.html

134) "NASA Study Finds World Warmth Edging Ancient Levels." September 25, 2006. Accessed December 31, 2009.
http://www.nasa.gov/vision/earth/
environment/world_warmth.html

135) Young., 75.

136) Castel, et al., xxi.

137) Wong, Cathy. What Are Goji Berries? August 1, 2006. Accessed February 14, 2010.
http://altmedicine.about.com/od/
completeazindex/a/goji.htm

LaVergne, TN USA
17 February 2011
216971LV00001B/85/P